Thomas Baldwin

Airopaidia

Containing the narrative of a balloon excursion from Chester, the eighth of September, 1785, taken from minutes made during the voyage: hints on the improvement of balloons, to which is subjoined mensuration of heights by the barometer

Thomas Baldwin

Airopaidia

Containing the narrative of a balloon excursion from Chester, the eighth of September, 1785, taken from minutes made during the voyage: hints on the improvement of balloons, to which is subjoined mensuration of heights by the barometer

ISBN/EAN: 9783337394837

Printed in Europe, USA, Canada, Australia, Japan

Cover: Foto ©ninafisch / pixelio.de

More available books at **www.hansebooks.com**

AIROPAIDIA:

CONTAINING

THE NARRATIVE OF A

BALLOON EXCURSION

from CHESTER, the eighth of September, 1785,
taken from MINUTES made DURING the Voyage:

H I N T S

ON THE IMPROVEMENT OF BALLOONS,
AND MODE OF INFLATION BY *STEAM:*
MEANS TO PREVENT THEIR DESCENT OVER WATER;
OCCASIONAL ENQUIRIES
INTO THE STATE OF THE ATMOSPHERE,
FAVOURING THEIR DIRECTION;
WITH VARIOUS PHILOSOPHICAL
OBSERVATIONS AND CONJECTURES.

TO WHICH IS SUBJOINED,
MENSURATION OF HEIGHTS BY THE BAROMETER,
MADE PLAIN:
WITH EXTENSIVE TABLES.

The WHOLE ſerving as an INTRODUCTION to

AËRIAL NAVIGATION:

WITH A COPIOUS INDEX.

BY THOMAS BALDWIN, ESQ. A. M.

- - - - - Addita NAVIGIIS ſunt
Multa.   *Lucretius De Rerum Nat.* L. 5, V. 335.
Nihil PERFECTUM ſimul ac INCEPTUM.

USUS UNI REI deditus, et NATURAM et ARTEM ſæpē
vincit.   *Cicero.*

C H E S T E R:

Printed for the Author, by J. Fletcher; and ſold by W.
Lowndes, No. 77, Fleet-ſtreet, London; J. Poole, Cheſter;
and other Bookſellers.

1786.
Price, in Boards, 7s. 6d.

TO THE

PRINCIPAL INHABITANTS

OF

CHESTER:

For their POLITE ATTENTION on the Day of Afcent, and Prefervation of ORDER during the INFLATION: on which, the Succefs of aërial Experiments fo much depends, and throu' the Want of which, fo many have already failed; for the kind Anxiety manifefted during his Abfence; and for their friendly CONGRATULATIONS, on his fafe Return; the following Account of the Balloon-Excurfion, written at their Requeft, is, by their Permiffion, with all Gratitude, Efteem and Refpect,

DEDICATED,

by their moft obliged,

and moft obedient Servant

THE AIRONAUT.

انجیلی

AN ACCOUNT OF THE PLATES; WITH DIRECTIONS FOR PLACING THEM.

1st. *An Account of the Plates.*

1. (*a*) A *Circular View from the Balloon at its greatest Elevation*, (Page 58.) The Spectator is supposed to be in the Car of the Balloon, suspended above the *Center* of the View: looking *down* on the Amphitheatre or *white* Floor of Clouds, and seeing the *City of Chester*, as it appeared throu' the *Opening*: which discovers the Landscape *below*, limited, by surrounding Vapour, to something less than *two* Miles in Diameter.

The Breadth of the *blue* Margin *defines* the *apparent* Height of the Spectator in the Balloon (viz. 4 Miles) *above* the *white* Floor of Clouds, as he hangs in the Center, and looks *horizontally* round, into the *azure* Sky.

2. (*b*) *The Balloon over Helsbye-Hill in Cheshire*, at half past II. on Thursday the 8th of September, 1785. (Page 78.)

It is seen in the *South-west-Quarter*.

The View was taken in a *high* Field, at the End of Sutton-Causeway.

Helsbye-Hill, tho' upwards of 600 *Feet high*, appeared from the Car of the Balloon, to be on the *same Level* with the *Grounds below*.

3. (*c*) *A Balloon-Prospect from above the Clouds*, (Page 154,) or *Chromatic* View of the Country between Chester, Warrington and Rixton-Moss in Lancashire: shewing the whole Extent of the aërial Voyage; with the *meandering* Track of the Balloon throu' the Air.

4. *The*

4. *The Explanatory Print* (*d*), (Page 155:) which elucidates the former by giving the Names of the principal Places mentioned in the Excursion.

N. B. *The Circular View* is seen to the best Advantage, when placed *flat* on a Table or Chair, and *rather* in the Shade: the Eye looking *directly* down upon the Picture.

Whoever will be at the Trouble of viewing *distinct* Parts of *the Balloon-Prospect*, throu' a very small Opening, made by rolling a Sheet of Paper into the Form of a hollow Tube, and applying it close to either Eye, at the same Time shutting the other; or by looking throu' the Hand, held a little open, and close to the Eye; may form a very accurate Idea of the Manner, in which the *Prospect below* was represented *gradually in Succession*, to the Aironaut; whose Sight was bounded by a Circularity of Vapour, as in Section 79, 221.

2d. *Directions for placing them.*

Place the *Top* of the CIRCULAR VIEW, *even* with the *Top* of the Page.

The Plate will then lye over at the Bottom, and at the *right* Side of the Page.

Fold the Bottom up into the Book, even with the Margin: and the *right* Side in like Manner.

Observe to place the *Bottom* of each of the other Plates, even with the *Bottom* of the Page.

The Plate will then lye *over* at the Top, and at the *right* Side of the Page.

Fold the Top *down*, into the Book, *even* with the Margin: and the right Side, in like Manner.

The circular View, to *face* Page 58.

The Balloon over Helſbye-Hill, to *face* Page 78.

The Balloon Proſpect, to *face* Page 154.

The explanatory Print, to be placed *on* Page 155: and, when unfolded, to be ſeen *along with* the Balloon-Proſpect.

(VII)

Literal and other Errors proper to be examined, and corrected with the Pen, before the Book is read.

Page.
6. Note *(a)*—ειαδεν write ευδαεν.
18. Note *(a)*—*Cube* of the Velocity, &c. *write* (as in some Copies) Square of the Velocity, &c. the Resistence will be as $3 \times 3 = 9$.—See Chambers's Dictionary, under RESISTENCE.
23. Section 21. *Blot out* [Signs] of Currents.
26. *Before* All Things being thus prepared, *insert* [Section] *viz.* 25.
35. Line 13.—I o'Clock, *write* I. o'Clock.
54. Section 52.—an Extent above them of 77 Miles, *write* an Extent of 102 Miles. See the Occasion of this Mistake in Note *(a)* Calculation SECOND, which makes the Answer 102 Miles, 1 Quarter, 320 Yards; and the Ans. to the
PROBLEM being 102   1 .   307
gives the Prospect - - - 13 Yards less than *that* over the Clouds.
84. Line 4.—great Turnpike-Road, *write* great public Road.
84. Note *(b)*. *After* See Moore's Practical Navigator, *insert* See Page 98 *(c)*.
98. *After* Note *(c) add* See Section 84, Note *(b)*.
118. Line 5.—from a vertical Situation only, to be seen, *write* to be seen from a vertical Situation only :.
174. Line 1.—excessine Diminution *write* excessive Diminution.
177. Line 9.—contain *write* contains.
202. The Sections 259, 260, 261, are repeated.
234. Line 6.—a Yard. *write* two Yards.
236. Line 3. *After the Words* in Danger of breaking; *add* the Bottom of the Balloon must be opened, or the upper Valve drawn. *And erase the Remainder of the Sentence.*
237. Line 4.—which is a Sign that the Balloon defcends, *write* (which is a Sign that the Balloon defcends).
242. Line 21.—supercede, *write* supersede.
263. Line 5.—commonly : ascend, *write* commonly ascend :.
266. Line 21.—their Passage *write* its Passage.
271. Line 14.—each 4 Feet *write* each 4 Inches.
278. Lines 15 and 18.—third Tables *and* third Table, *write* fourth Tables *and* fourth Table.
283. Note *(a)*.—more than the three first Decimals *write* more than the four first Decimals.
288. Line 5. *After* .0000076, *insert* which, being divided by .1, gives a Cypher less.
288. Line 11.—with 4° on .25, *write* with 4° on 25.

290. Note

(VIII)

290. Note *(a)*—at low Water.) *write* at low Water.
292. Line 23.—there will remain the greater Height, *write* there will remain, SECONDLY; (see Section 367) the greater Height.
303. Line 6.—(viz. the 8,) *write* (viz. the .8,).
309. Line 10. Marginal Note.—*7th Step in Section 366.* write *7th Step in Section 368.*
310. *After* Line 23, *insert Air.* Thermom. 56°.
311. Line 1.—By the Practice of the first Example, *write* Practice of the second Example.
312. Line 29. *After* The Answer, &c. *insert* , made by rejecting a Cypher,.
317. Before the last Line but two, *insert* END OF THE FIRST STAGE.
318. Line 23.—the 2d Tenth, *write* the 1st Tenth.
319. Line 13.— , gives 7. *write* , gives 97.
322. last Line but two.—and the remaining Feet *write* the remaining Feet.

AIROPAIDIA:
CHAPTER I.

Section 1. **THE** Public have, for *Introduction.* a confiderable Time, been entertained with Accounts of aërial Voyages.

Such Accounts are, in many Refpects, vague and unfatisfactory: by no Means adequate to the Expectations and Wifhes, which have been formed by thofe, who have not yet penetrated the profound Heights of the Atmofphere.

2. The Voyagers have, now and *Miftakes to be noticed, as Examples of Avoidance.* then, been pretty accurate in Regard to Time Place Diftance and Velocity: Circumftances highly worthy of Remark, in order to eftimate the Improvement already made in this wonderful Difcovery, and point out its Ufe: but neither ought the *feveral Occafions of Failure* in the Experiments

B   to

to be omitted; as they will be found to arise more from a Want of Prudence and Foresight in the Managers, than from any Defect in the Machine, or the Principle on which it acts. Such Failure ought therefore to throw an additional Light and Credit on the Art: and give a Spur to Ingenuity, which, it is not to be doubted, will continue to drive forwards with the same rapid Success; nor rest, till the Art itself is brought to the highest Degree of Perfection; till airostatic Ships make the Circuit of the Globe: a NAVIGATION which, from its Novelty and Importance, deserves to be considered in a separate Treatise.

Aërial Voyagers defective in their Descriptions.

3. Balloon-Voyagers have likewise been particularly defective in their Descriptions of aërial Scenes and Prospects: those Scenes of majestic Grandeur which the unnumbered Volumes of encircling Clouds, in most fantastic Forms and various Hues, beyond Conception glowing and transparent, portray

tray to a Spectator placed as in a Center of the Blue Serene above them: contemplating at the same Instant, and *apparently* at some Miles Distance immediately below, a most exquisite and ever-varying Miniature of the *little Works of Man*, heightened by the supreme Pencil of Nature, inimitably elegant, and in her highest Colouring.

Such are the Scenes which, Ballooners all allow, constitute the true Sublime and Beautiful: inspire Ideas of rational Humiliation to a thinking Mind, and raise the most careless Mortal to an unknown Degree of enthusiastic Rapture and Pleasure.

Every Beholder is a Judge of the Scenery around him; and no one, it is presumed, ever ascended into the Atmosphere on a *mild Day*, with a sound and well ballasted Balloon, that did not wish to taste the Luxury of a second Voyage.

4. Yet notwithstanding, as Ignorance is known to be the Parent of Fear, Disappointment shoud excite the Ardor of the Scientific.

Fear, the Bulk of Mankind, which are by far the greater Number, will long continue to entertain abſurd Apprehenſions concerning it; to oppoſe and ridicule the Invention; as they will oppoſe every other Diſcovery, which they have neither Talents *Inclination* or Leiſure to underſtand.

This Reflexion ſhoud, on the contrary, rather excite than check the Ardor of the Skilful and Scientific, to cheriſh and promote the Art.

In the Hiſtory of Airoſtation, each Event is yet new and *uncompared. Every* Circumſtance ought therefore to be carefully recorded: ſince it woud be unfair to fix Bounds to Science; or argue, that ſuch Inferences, as ſhall demonſtrate the great Utility of the Invention, may not be drawn from Circumſtances which Inattention might pronounce to be moſt trifling and minute.

The Reader cautioned.

5. The Reader is requeſted to obſerve that, this Account being addreſſed

dreſſed to the Generality, and not to the Curious and Philoſophic only; many Circumſtances are added, which woud otherwiſe have been conſidered as ſuperfluous: and ſome it was thought proper to repeat, in order to connect the Thread of the Narration, without the Neceſſity of frequent Reference to the Sections.

6. An Agreement having been made with Mr. Lunardi, that he ſhoud reſign his Balloon to Mr. Baldwin on Wedneſday the 7th of September; an Advertiſement to that Purpoſe appeared in the Cheſter Paper: and on Wedneſday Morning, a great Number of Spectators aſſembled in the Caſtle-yard of the City of Cheſter: where many waited till half paſt IV in the Afternoon; Mr. Lunardi declaring that, on Account of the Violence and Unſteadineſs of the Wind which blew from the South and South-Weſt, it was dangerous to attempt the Inflation of his Balloon; and Mr. Baldwin continuing

Squalls of Wind the Day preceding the Aſcent.

tinuing to assert that, if it coud be filled, he was willing to go up.

The Weather was *then* moderate: but Mr. Baldwin, thinking the Hour too late to begin the Inflation, which, judging from the two former Inflations, coud not probably have been completed till after *Sunset*; made a Proposal to Mr. Lunardi, that he shoud postpone the Exhibition till the next (*a*) Day. The latter, after some Reluctance, arising from a Fear lest the Public shoud disapprove his Conduct, politely complied with his Request, on Mr. Baldwin's saying that he woud take the Blame on himself.

CHAPTER

(*a*) Ποιησον δ' Αιθρην, δος δ' Οφθαλμοῖσιν ιδεσθαι·
Ἐν δε Φαει και ολεσσον, επει νυ τοι ειαδεν ἐτως.
    Homer's Iliad, Book 17, Line 646.

CHAPTER II.

Preparations for the Voyage.

Section 7. ON Thursday the 8th of September 1785, at IX in the Morning, one of the Cannons (a Six-pounder) was first fired in the Castle-yard, to inform the City and Neighbourhood, that the necessary Preparations were making to inflate the Balloon. *Cannon first fired at IX.*

Till VIII that Morning, the Air had been hazy: but was then clear, bright and calm *below*, with an upper Tier of light Clouds in the Zenith moving from South-West by West, and dense ones rising in the Horizon.

8. At X o'Clock, the Process began with the Inflation of an airostatic Globe eighteen Feet in Circumference, of Silk Tiffany, made the latter End of the Year 1783, and decorated with Painting, Mottoes and Devices: in the *At X, the Inflation began with a small Balloon.*

the Performance of which little Work, Mr. Baldwin was (in the modern Phrase) the sole Projector, Architect Workman and Chymist.

An airostatic Globe liberated as Pioneer to the great one. 9. The Airostat was presently liberated by the Hands of Mr. Lunardi; and continuing to turn gently the same Way round its own Axis, afforded a beautiful Spectacle to the Beholders: remaining in Sight about half an Hour. It was intended to serve as a Sort of Pioneer, to delineate the Track of the great Balloon.

Its Fate. 10. It fell at some Miles Distance, 'tis said unfortunately on a Hedge, and was presently torn to Pieces by the Eagerness and Avarice of the Pursuers, who expected and undeservedly obtained the Reward promised in the Letter appended to it.

Second Cannon, at XII. 11. At XII the Cannon fired a second Time, to announce that the Process was in a proper Degree of Forwardness.

At

At this Time Mr. Baldwin went, with some Friends, to take an early Dinner: he also recapitulated the Articles, to be certain that Nothing was omitted.

12. The following Inventory, with which he ascended, may be of Use to future Aironauts; to whom *only* it is addressed.

<small>Inventory for the Voyage.</small>

The Cable and Grapple are considered as Part of the Balloon. (See Section 13.)

12. Article 1. A portable Barometer, *(a)* with a common Syphon or Bulb, (purchased at Lausanne.)

12. 2. Martin's Thermometer, *(b)* with Farenheit's Scale *(c)* for the Degrees of Temperature.

12. 3. Com-

(a) Phil. Transf. Vol. LXVII, for 1777, Part II, Page 513, containing Sir G. Shuckburgh's Rules for the Mensuration of Heights with the Barometer. Also Vol. LXVIII, for 1778, Part II, Page 681:

(b) And Page 688.

(c) It were to be wished that the Divisions of the Thermometer by Farenheit were become general throughout Europe, in preference to those by Reaumur yet retained *abroad*; which Divisions of Reaumur are not sufficiently minute to mark the least sensible Change in the Temperature, are subject to frequent Mistakes, and the Inconvenience of adding in the Notation, the Words *above* or *below* the Cypher, zero, or Point of Congelation: besides their being in Conversation not easily compared with those of Farenheit; each Degree of the latter having to that of the former nearly the Proportion of 18 to 11: since Farenheit from the freezing Point upwards to boiling Water has $212-32=180°$, and Reaumur to the same Height,

INVENTORY FOR THE VOYAGE

12. 3. Mariner's Compaſs in a double Box, to be uſed when the Sun is intercepted from the View by Clouds, in order to diſcover whether the Balloon turns round.

12. 4. Down, or ſmall Feathers, to be looſe in the Pocket, and thrown out, when enſhrined in Clouds; or at any other Time, to ſhew the Riſe or Fall of the Balloon.

12. 5. An Aſſes' Skin Patent Pocket-book; as Wet ſpoils Paper.

12. 6. Two *red* Lead Pencils: each Pencil ready pointed at both Ends, to ſave Time and Trouble: preferable to Ink, which may be ſpilt or frozen.

The Strokes with *red* Lead are not ſo eaſily obliterated, as when made with a *black* Lead Pencil.

12. 7. A ſmall ſharp Knife pointed, and ready open, or which will open eaſily. A Pair of Sciſſars.

12. 8. A

110° Diviſions: Mr. Sauſſure ſays as 4 to 9; in which there is an evident Overſight: ſee his curious and philoſophic Inveſtigation of the Atmoſphere in "Eſſais ſur L'Hygrometrie." 4to. A Neuchatel, 1783.

Frequent Mention being made of the Thermometer graduated according to Farenheit's Scale, in different Parts of the following Account; it may not be amiſs to ſhew the correſponding Points according to Reaumur, taken from "Thermometre univerſel de Comparaiſon, extrait du Journal de Phyſique de M. L'Abbé Rozier."

Farenheit.				Reaumur.
54	-	-	-	13 & 4-9ths above the Cypher.
55	-	-	-	14 ditto, nearly.
57	-	-	-	15 2-9ths ditto, nearly.
59	-	-	-	16 4-9ths ditto, nearly.
60	-	-	-	17 1-9th ditto.
65	-	-	-	20 1-9th ditto, nearly.

12. 8. A *wicker* Bottle of Brandy and Water, only three Parts full, half and half: such Bottles are more secure: and such Mixture will not soon freeze. The cochuc or elastic Bottle is still better. A Cork-screw.

12. 9. *Compact* Provisions, which do not soil the Fingers or Pocket-book, as Confectionaries, Fruit, Biscuit, Bread.

12. 10. A *boarded* Map of the Country over which the Aironaut may be supposed to pass: the Back serving as a Table.

12. 11. Two Needles with large Eyes: the *raw* Silk put through, and tyed on a Knot at the Ends to prevent the Needles from being lost: to be ready at the Instant wanted, to sew up any Holes within Reach, in the Balloon; the Holes being first tyed up with Twine.

The Needles to be stuck into Parchment, containing a small Hank of *raw* Silk: the Needle Silk run round the Parchment, to keep the Hank dry.

The whole Hank to be tyed by one End to the Side of the Car; when above all Clouds, to shew, by the Divergency of the Threads, the Electricity of the Air.

12. 12. A few Yards of Dutch Twine, loose in the Pocket, to tye the Neck of the Balloon in descending.

12. 13. For easy Experiments; 1st, Dutch Twine, half a Mile long, on a Reel, or Pulley, or two Lengths on different Reels: also to each

Reel

Reel a Flag, made of white Linen, a Yard square; and ſtretched by a ſlender Lath; one Side of the Flag being bound and ſtitched round it: alſo a Piece of Twine, two Yards long, is to be faſtened by its Ends to the Ends of the Lath: a Loop is to be made in the Middle of the Twine: and to the Loop is to be applied round the Middle of the Lath another Piece of Twine, which will prevent the Lath from being bent; and will keep the Flag always ſtretched.

By this Apparatus, Obſervers from below may be enabled to eſtimate the Height of the Balloon, as will be ſhewn in its proper Place.

12. 14. 2dly, To try the Denſity of the Air, at different Heights, *above* the freezing Point with Water; *below* it, with Brandy.

In a Baſket take two Pint-bottles, one full of Water, the other of Brandy; and ſix or eight empty ones: alſo a ſmall Metal Tunning-diſh.

Let one End of a String be tyed round the Neck of each Bottle: and the other End ſealed to the Top of a large Cork much tapered, to enter the Mouth eaſily. Round each Neck, tye a Parchment Label, large enough to contain in abbreviated Characters the Number of the Bottle; Time of Obſervation, Heights of the Barometer and Thermometer, while on the Ground.

When an Experiment is made in the Air; pour off a full Bottle into an empty one: put the Cork into the emptied Bottle, and mark again the
Time,

Time, Barometer and Thermometer: which are to be compared with an Eudiometer below, to difcover the Rarity and Purity of the Atmofphere.

12. 15. A third white Linen Flag, made as above, and tyed to the upper Hoop of the Balloon, fo as to hang in Sight, will give Notice of a Change in the Wind.

12. 16. A Yard of thin Ribbon, two Inches broad, tyed to the lower Hoop, will mark the Rife and Fall of the Balloon.

(12. 17. A Magnet and Iron Filings in a thin Pewter Difh with a Cover; Alfo

The Prifm and large Telefcope were left, as too heavy.) And the Sextant or Quadrant coud not be procured in Time. They woud have been of little Ufe, as no Horizon of the round Earth was feen during the Excurfion: and it is prefumed, that the circular Horizon is feldom vifible, when the Balloon is at any confiderable Height; the Accumulation of Vapour between the Eye and Horizon preventing it: tho' fuch Vapour remains invifible to Spectators from below.

12. 18. Eight Bladders, each above half blown, and differently coloured for Ornament, tyed round the *upper* Part of the Car, Breaft high when the Aironaut ftands upright: in Cafe the Balloon fall into Water.

12. 19. Speaking Trumpet: alfo a live Pigeon, in a fmall Bafket of Matting.

12. 20. Pep-

12. 20. Pepper, Salt, Ginger; to try the Effects of Tastes, which have been said to become insipid on the Peak of Teneriffe.

CHAPTER III.

ADDRESSED TO AIRONAUTS.

New Kind of Cable and Reel recommended.

Section 13. THE following Anchor and Cable, for greater Safety and some particular Uses, are recommended as an Improvement.

A *strong* Iron double Grapple, moving on a Swivel, fastened to a *Rope*, (*a*) half

(*a*) The Strength of the Rope, or Cable, if its Length does not exceed 10 or 12 Yards, ought to be such as to support a weight, greater than the Weight of the Balloon and it's Appendages, for the Resistance made by the Grapple against the Balloon acted on by the Wind is immediate: The Rope ought therefore to be made of Indian-Gut, as most elastic, or Silk, as lightest. But if the Rope be half a Mile, or a Mile long; the Resistance is gradual: the Balloon descending for some Minutes; and having an open Space to move in through the Air: the Rope or Cable acting as a Radius, and the Levity of the Balloon and Opposition of the circumambient Air preventing it from falling with any Violence.

The shorter Cable may be used at the Height

half a Mile, or better *a Mile* long: and, if not all; a Part of which at leaſt, at the Diſtance and for the Length of ten Yards from the Grapple, ſhoud be of Silk, as a non Conductor: alſo other ten Yards, at its upper End, counting from the Reel or Pulley to which the Silk ſhoud be tyed.

The Reel or Pulley being at leaſt eighteen Inches in Diameter, and fixed vertically in the Center of the upper Hoop, ſeven Feet above the Bottom of the Car; by Means of three or four Iron Rods faſtened in the Bottom of the Car, and meeting together above the Reel: the Rods ſo ſtrong as to prevent the Shock which otherwiſe the Aironaut woud receive in alighting on the Ground.

The Reel ſhoud have one, or two Iron Winches or Handles, one at each End of the Reel; with moveable Handles of 10 Yards; in aid of the longer, to prevent it from riſing; or to moor it, by winding the Reel, and hauling down the Balloon cloſe to the Ground.

CAUTIONS TO BE OBSERVED.

Handles of Wood round them. The Reel may be furnished with sudden Checks; or gradual Clamps, as in a Mill, to retard the Velocity.

SIGNS TO BE OBSERVED, WHEN IN THE AIR.

Cautions against two Extremes.

14. The two Extremes to be avoided are, too lofty an Ascent: and too precipitate a Fall.

1st, Too lofty an Ascent.

The former is to be apprehended when the Balloon has swelled considerably, and strains as if ready to burst: from the Shape of an inverted Cone, or Children's Top, changed to that of an oblate Spheroid, or Turnep.

It is therefore necessary to look up at the Balloon from Time to Time: and either open the Mouth, or as it is sometimes called the Neck, *for an Instant*; or draw the Valve; which is done by pulling a Cord fixed at the Top of the Machine and running thro' it to the Hand, till the Balloon only appears full without straining.

These Operations are to be occasionally repeated during the *Ascent*.

CAUTIONS TO BE OBSERVED.

If it is required to rife ftill higher; gradually throw out Ballaft, and repeat the Operations.

The propofed Quantity of Ballaft being thrown out, the Balloon will have acquired its utmoft Height, and become ftationary, i. e. neither rife nor fall.

The felf Defcent of the Balloon is only in Proportion, as the inflammable Air or Gafs efcapes thro' imperceptible Holes in the Silk or Seams.

2dly. TO PREVENT TOO PRECIPITATE A FALL.

15. 1ft. Tye, or comprefs the Mouth of the Balloon, for a Moment; which muft always be opened, on obferving that the Balloon is again rifen to fo great a Height as to *ftrain*, or be diftended as above mentioned.

2dly. Caution againft too precipitate a Fall.

2d. In defcending, throw out Ballaft, when the Balloon is within a Quarter of a Mile of the Ground, but not before, i. e. at 26 Inches by the Barometer: and, if the Fall is precipitate

tate, not lefs than 25 Pounds Averdupoife, Pound by Pound, or at once, if there fhould be Occafion.

3d. In Cafe of Accident, as the Efcape of Gafs; or if the Balloon be not furnifhed with AN EQUATORIAL HOOP; prepare to throw out all the Ballaft at the above Height, but not before; as the more forcible the Fall, *(a)* the greater the *Refiftance* from the Air: cut away Ends of Cords; tear off Ornaments: part with Shoes, Cloaths. All which muft be made *loofe* and *ready* to throw out, at the Moment the Balloon begins to defcend. Before the Landing, particular Care muft be taken, that the Weight of the Aironaut be fuftained, by grafping the Hands round the OPPOSITE Sides of the upper Hoop; fo that the Feet may not touch the Bottom of the Car. The Knees fhoud likewife be bent.

(a) The Refiftance being as the Cube of the Velocity; therefore if the Velocity be increafed 3 Times, the Refiftance will be as $3 \times 3 = 9$, i. e. will be increafed 9 Times.

bent. Repeating the above, at each Rebound of the Balloon, if any; the Aironaut will alight in the gentleſt Manner: and probably the Balloon may act as a Paraſhute or Umbrella; which *alone* will, at all Times, enſure an eaſy Deſcent.

SIGNS WHEREBY TO JUDGE WHETHER THE BALLOON IS RISING OR FALLING.

SIGNS OF RISING.

16. 1. When the Aironaut perceives a Preſſure upwards againſt the Soles of his Feet. Signs of Aſcent or Deſcent.

2. When ſome Objects, on the Surface of the Earth immediately below, diminiſh, and others diſappear.

3. When an upper Cloud approaches or involves the Balloon.

4. When a lower Cloud leaves the Balloon.

5. When Rain Snow or Hail beat VIOLENTLY againſt the Top of the Balloon.

6. When

6. When Feathers, Balloon-Flag, or Ribbon seem to be drawn forcibly downwards.

7. When Objects on Earth, or among Clouds below the Balloon, rise and present themselves *beyond those*, which, the moment before, were thought most distant.

8. When the Balloon appears broader and shorter; also fuller at the Bottom; being more distended than at the first Ascent.

SIGNS OF DESCENT.

<small>Signs of Descent.</small>

17. 1. When the Aironaut perceives the Bottom of the Car withdrawing itself from the Pressure against the Soles of his Feet.

2. When Objects on Earth, and surrounding Prospects encrease in Magnitude and Number.

3. When a lower Cloud approaches or involves the Balloon.

4. When an upper Cloud leaves the Balloon.

5. When

5. When Weather beats against the Bottom of the Car or Balloon.

6. When Feathers, Balloon-Flag, or Ribbon appear to be drawn upwards.

7. When the most distant Objects *set,* and disappear.

8. When the Balloon seems taller; and its lower Hemisphere less distended, tho' continuing *tight*.

SIGNS OF PROGRESSIVE HORIZONTAL MOTION.

18. These are equivocal and deceitful. When the Aironaut has lost Sight of the Earth by intervening Clouds; the Balloon seems at Rest, and only the lower Clouds appear to move: whereas the contrary may be true, the Clouds may rest, and only the Balloon move.

In this Case, Attention must be paid to the half Mile white Flag, whose Situation and Motion must be observed, with respect to the Balloon, and

to

Signs of progressive Motion deceitful.

to the Earth before the Cloud intervened. If the Flag retains its Situation with Respect to the Balloon, it may be inferred that no Change in the Direction has happened: if its Situation alters, the Sun or Compass is to be observed: and an Estimate made of the new Current of Air by which the Balloon is affected: its Velocity, Sound, Temperature, &c.

To descend when lost. 19. But to acquire a Certainty of the Course, it will be proper to descend below the Cloud: or move by Compass, Map, and a Knowledge of the Country: or try the long Cable (Section 13.)

Signs of Wind horizontal. 20. It is likewise necessary to know the *Signs of Wind,* or Currents of Air.

SIGNS OF NEW AND SUDDEN HORIZONTAL CURRENTS.

When the Feathers, Balloon-Flag, or Ribbon, compared with Sun or Compass, take a new and sudden horizontal Direction.

21. SIGNS

21. SIGNS OF CURRENTS FROM ABOVE: properly named *Waves Torrents and Tide of Air.*

[margin: Signs of depressing Torrents and Tide of Air.]

They are very frequent, and require to be guarded againſt: are ſometimes of long Continuance, at other Times momentary: againſt the firſt throw out Ballaſt at the Height of a Quarter of a Mile, but not before, or *as hereafter directed:* when momentary, and above that Height, Nothing is to be apprehended: the Balloon will appear broader and recover its Form.

CHAPTER IV.

PREPARATIONS FOR ASCENT.

Section 22. BEFORE half paſt I, Mr. Lunardi had inflated his Balloon in the fineſt Manner; and having, with the moſt obliging and ſpirited Attention, made

[margin: Preparations for Aſcent.]

ſuch

such Preparations, and taken such Preparations, as he thought were neceſſary to enſure the Succeſs of the Expedition; ſent to inform Mr. Baldwin (who continued purpoſely abſent, that he might not diſturb or precipitate the Proceſs; but that every Circumſtance ſhoud be conducted with Deliberation and without Hurry) that all Things were ready for his Departure.

The Public reminded of the Neceſſity of preſerving Order during the Inflation of Balloons.

23. And Mr. Baldwin takes this Opportunity of returning his beſt Thanks to his Friends and the Public, on the Day of Aſcent, for keeping THE SMALL CIRCLE CLEAR, by ſtrictly adhering to the Words of the Advertiſement, which declared, " that in order to prevent an Interruption of the Proceſs in the Inflation of the Balloon, no Perſons *were* to be admitted WITHIN THE CIRCLE, except thoſe Gentlemen who politely undertook IN TURN to hold the Lines which detained the Balloon."

24. It

PREPARATIONS FOR THE VOYAGE. 25

24. It may be proper to mention that Mr. Baldwin being resolved to prevent the disagreeable Circumstances of being *weighed* in the Presence of some Thousand Spectators, at a Time when it is uncertain whether the Balloon has *acquired* a sufficient Degree of Levity to raise his own Weight, together with the Instruments, Provisions, Ballast, and other Articles, all which are known or easily calculated; finding some Days before, his own Weight, and having calculated the rest as under (*a*); he ordered his Servant, on the Day of the Excursion, to bring Lead Weights equal to the *Sum total,* with an overplus Weight of 10lb. for Levity of Ascent, and place them *gradually* in the Car, attached for that Purpose

Lead Weights placed at first in the Car, to prevent any Fatigue in holding the Lines, and the Necessity of weighing, unless at the Time of Ascent, to determine the Power of Levity.

	Pounds Averdupois.
(*a*) Weight of the Aironaut	160
Provisions and Articles calculated at	20
Sand-Ballast prepared in Bags	44
Levity for Ascent	10
Sum total,	234

Purpose to the Balloon, soon after the Inflation began. By which Means the Gentlemen who held the Cords were quite at Ease: nor was there Occasion to tye the Lines during the Inflation, to Posts fixed in the Circumference of the Circle; nor consequently to *cut them* afterwards.

But it will be seen that Mr. Lunardi inflated the Balloon in a superior Manner.

All Things being thus prepared, Mr. Baldwin stepped into the Car: and finding, that, besides his own Weight, the Provisions, Articles, Ballast, &c. the Balloon woud support an additional Weight, and *still* rise with superior Levity; Mr. Lunardi put in 12lb. of additional Ballast, and *guessed* the encreased Levity at 10lb. more.

$$
\begin{array}{r}
\text{Additional} \begin{cases} \text{Ballast} & - - \ 12 \\ \text{Levity} & - - \ 10 \end{cases} \\
\overline{22} \\
\text{Added to the } 234 \\
\overline{\text{Make the Sum } 256\text{lb.}}
\end{array}
$$

All

All which added to the Weight of the Balloon, *by Information only*, as follows:

Balloon varnished - -	113
Netting and Cords - -	18
Car and Hoops - - -	24
Mended and added Parts -	5
Grapple and Cable - -	4
	164
With the	256

Make the total Levity of the Gafs to produce an Equilibrium, equal to - - - - - - - - 420lb.

The Weight of a Quantity of Air equal in Bulk to the Balloon, being fecluded; and the Gafs fubftituted in its Room.

26. The Calculation of the Weight of Articles was, as follows:

Weight of Articles.

Articles.	Pounds Averd.	Ounces.
1. Eight coloured Bladders (*a*) (Section 13, Art. 18)	1	0
2. Preparations againft extreme Cold. A WINTER DRESS. Flannel or woollen Socks ⎫ Cap -. - - - - - ⎪ Gloves - - - - - ⎬ Drawers - - - - ⎪ Under Stockings - - ⎪ ——— Waiftcoat - - ⎭	0	14

3. Brandy

(*a*) Ancient Warriors among the Arabs, Spaniards, Romans, Gauls, and Germans, being frequently obliged to pafs deep Rivers, never undertook a Campaign without them. For the above Anecdote, and many curious Experiments on Air, fee Sam. Reyheri, *Differtatio de Aëre*, tertium edita. Kiliæ. 1673.

3. Brandy, Water, Flask, and Refreshments - - -	1	8
4. Barometer (portable) - -	0	$12\frac{1}{2}$
5. Thermometer - - - -	0	3
6. Dial-Compass (a Mariner's Compass in a double Box, will traverse better) - -	0	$3\frac{1}{2}$
7. Two white Flags, with Dutch Twine on two Reels furnished with Swivels - - - - -	0	4
	2	8
8. Asses Skin Pocket Book, Blank Cards, Pencils, Knife and Scissars - -	0	$4\frac{1}{2}$
9. Map of Cheshire boarded, the superfluous Parts cut away - - - - - -	0	3
10. Speaking Trumpet - -	0	$8\frac{1}{2}$
11. Mr. Lunardi's Flag - -	3	8
12. Basket and eight Pint Bottles labelled, one full of Brandy, another of Water	8	3
	20	0

Weight of Ballast.

27. The Ballast consisted of three Bags of dry Sand, and two red grit Stones, taken while in the Car, *additional.*

1st Bag tyed up weighed - - -	12lb.
2d Ditto - - - - - -	12
3d untyed Ditto - - - -	20
1st red Grit - - - - -	7
2d red Grit - - - - -	5
In all	56lb.

CHAPTER V.

ASCENT WITH 20lb. OF LEVITY.

Section 28. AT 40 Minutes past I, the Balloon having a Levity which not less than 20 Pounds Weight woud counterpoise, Mr. Baldwin was liberated by the Hands of Mr. Lunardi, who suffered no one to approach the Car: and he ascended, amidst Acclamations mixed with Tears of Delight and Apprehension, the Misgivings of Humanity, and other usual Sensations of Surprize, which, in a brilliant and numerous Assembly, will long continue to accompany a Spectacle so novel interesting and awful, as that of seeing a Fellow Mortal separated in a Moment from the Earth, and rushing to the Skies. *Ascent at 40M. past I, with 20lb. of Levity.*

29. The Balloon well inflated, tower'd aloft in an upright and perpendicular *Employments of the Aironaut.*

cular Direction, with a quick Motion, and an accelerated Velocity.

The Aironaut having ftood up, for a Minute or two, waving his Hat in the left, and faluting the Spectators with Mr. Lunardi's coloured Flag in the right Hand; put on his Hat, and having faftened the Flag-Staff horizontally among the Lines of the Balloon, immediately betook himfelf to different Employments, before he woud indulge in looking over the Brink of the Car; left the Novelty of the Profpect fhoud call off his Attention from *Things of Moment.*

Senfation of rifing defcribed. 30. The Force of Afcent was, from the firft, plainly *palpable:* the Senfation being that of a ftrong Preffure from the Bottom of the Car, upwards againft the Soles of the Feet.

Caution againft the vitriolic Acid Liquor. 31. His firft Point being to guard againft a Deluge of acidulous Liquor, which, he was told, had fallen, to the Quantity of three Quarts, on the Head and Shoulders of a former Aironaut,

naut, from the Trunk or Bottom of the Balloon, which ended in a wide circular Opening of eighteen Inches Diameter; he found that when the Weight either of himself, or of the Ballaft, was not exactly in the Center of the Car; the Opening of the Balloon woud, without any Trouble, hang so as to lie on the Outfide of the Car: but he did not perceive more than a few Drops iffue from the Mouth: which happened a few Minutes after he arofe.

32. This Difficulty vanifhing; he changed his erect into an inclined Pofture between fitting and kneeling; fometimes with the right Knee near the Bottom and Center of the Car: and having both Hands quite free, the Balloon being fubject to no *fenfible Motion*; he reconnoitred all the Lines and Cords: coiled the Rope or Cable to which the Anchor or grappling Iron was fixed: tyed faft its proper End to the upper Hoop: obferved and felt the superior

Attitude, and farther Employments.

superior Thickness of the Cord leading to the Valve: coiled it, in order that it might be free to act: placed the untyed Bag of Ballast near the Outside of the Car: also the tyed Bags at proper Distances to preserve the Equilibrium: unwrapped one of the white Flags, tyed it to the String on one of the Reels, and just threw it an Inch or two over the Side of the Car: then placed his Watch, *open* Knife, Scissars, Thermometer and Compass on his right Hand: the Barometer being swung above in Sight towards the left.

Change of Attitude, and Observation of the reddish Vapour. 33. He then stood on his Feet, with a Design to look down: but his Attention was drawn to the Opening of the Balloon, which began to breathe out by Intervals a visible *reddish Vapour*; in Form like that which is seen at the Top of a Brewery, only that the under Surface was not jagged but smooth, altho' wavy and uneven. The Particles which composed it were so large as to be distinctly visible: and appeared, ed, as if endued with a very ſtrong repelling Power, from the great and ſeemingly equal Diſtances, of about half a Quarter of an Inch, from each other.

It was obſerved by a ſcientific Spectator from below, that the Parts of the Balloon, which reflected the Sun's Rays, appeared of a bright Copper-Colour: but the *reddiſh* Vapour iſſuing from its Mouth put on the Form of a lambent Flame. A ſimilar Appearance had been obſerved by him, in a former Aſcent of the ſame Balloon, the Neck or Mouth being then likewiſe open; and alſo by others, who declared they ſaw the Balloon on Fire.

The Change of the RED into Flame-Colour, when ſeen at a great Diſtance, may it not be owing to this, that the direct Rays, being mingled with thoſe which are intercepted between the Eye and the Object, became in Part abſorbed,

The Gafs not offenfive.

34. This gentle Evaporation of inflammable Air, or Gafs, continued: difappearing at the Diftance of four and five Inches below the Opening: nor did it offend the Smell; not defcending within its Influence.

Attention to the Balloon, and Dimenfions of the Car and Hoops.

35. He then looked upwards at the Balloon, and perceived that it was confiderably fwelled in its Dimenfions: and that the Diftention had raifed the Bottom-Opening of the Balloon half way between the two Hoops: i. e. from his Hip to his Shoulder, as he ftood upright. The Height from the Bottom of the Car (which was a thin circular Board four Feet and a half, Diameter, placed on a ftrong Netting, and covered with green Bays) to its Top or the lower Hoop, was three Feet; with the Netting continued round between the lower and upper Hoop.

Stationary, and Notes made.

36. He was aware that the Swelling of the Balloon, and copious Vapour
then

then issuing from it, denoted the Moment when it began to lose its ascensional or elevating Power; and that its accelerated Motion was diminishing.

He therefore looked at his Barometer and Watch, which was 53 Minutes past I. *(a)*; took up his Pencil, and on a Card (marked before he left the Earth, as follows:

Chester-Castle-Yard. Thursday, the 8th of Sept. 1785, I. o'Clock, Barometer $29\frac{8}{10}$, Therm: 65 in the Shade towards the North;) he wrote " Rose at 40 Minutes past I." He then looked again at the Barometer, which continued falling for some Minutes, and fluctuating up and down within the Space of an Inch or more. It first began to rest at $23\frac{1}{4}$, and a little after at $23\frac{1}{2}$. Having looked again at his Watch, he put down " 57 Minutes past I. became stationary: Barometer $23\frac{1}{4}$: Therm:

(a) Equal Time with a Regulator corrected by an Observation.

Therm: still 65, sometimes lying in the Shade, and sometimes exposed to the Sun: the Balloon turning round frequently thro' East to South."

Fluctuation of Barometer,

37. The Fluctuation of the Barometer he imagined to arise from continued Exertions of the Gafs within the Balloon, opposed by the atmospheric Air, which varying in Density and Temperature woud give an unequal Resistance to the Balloon: and both Gafs and Air being elastic, the Power of Ascent would act by Intervals, and communicate its Pulsations to the Quicksilver in the Tube. His own irregular Motions in the Car would increase the Fluctuation.

The Compafs traverfed, but was ufelefs.

38. The Compafs likewife traversed backwards and forwards, pointing due North, and unaffected by the Turns of the Balloon: but was useless, as the Sun shone bright the whole Time of the Excursion. *(a)*

39. Things

(*a*) Being a Dial-Compafs, the Dipping of the Needle was frequently checked by the Glafs at the Top. A Mariner's Compafs is the beft.

39. Things taking a favourable Turn, he ſtood up, but with Knees a little bent, more eaſily to conform to accidental Motions, as Sailors when they walk the Deck: and took a full Gaze before, and below him. *Aironaut firſt looked down at Leiſure.*

But what Scenes of Grandeur and Beauty! *Scenes below deſcribed.*

A Tear of pure Delight flaſhed in his Eye! of pure and exquiſite Delight and Rapture; to look down on the unexpected Change already wrought in the Works of Art and Nature, con‑ tracted to a Span by the NEW PER‑ SPECTIVE, diminiſhed almoſt beyond the Bounds of Credibility.

Yet ſo far were the Objects from loſing their Beauty, that EACH WAS BROUGHT UP in a new Manner to the Eye, and dif‑ tinguiſhed by a Strength of Colouring, a Neatneſs and Elegance of Boundary, above Deſcription charming!

The endleſs Variety of Objects, minute, diſtinct and ſeparate, tho' ap‑ parently on the ſame Plain or Level, at once ſtriking the Eye without a Change

of its Pofition, aftonifhed and enchant-
ed. Their Beauty was unparalelled.
The Imagination itfelf was more than
gratified; *it was overwhelmed.*

The gay Scene was Fairy-Land,
and Chefter Lilliput.

He tried his Voice, and fhouted for
Joy. His Voice was unknown to
himfelf, fhrill and feeble.

There was no Echo.

<small>Let down the white Flag, 2 Furlongs, equal to half the Length of the Twine on one Reel.</small>

40. He then returned to an Employment which, tho' irkfome, he
imagined would contribute to the A-
mufement and Information of Spectators below, if it coud be completed

<small>Its Ufes.</small>

while he continued in Sight; as it
woud furnifh them with Ideas of
Height and Diftance, altogether new
and interefting, *as will be feen in their
proper Place:* and unwound half the
Reel; the white Flag hanging out to
the Length of 440 Yards or a Quarter
of a Mile.

<small>The Reel de-fective.</small>

41. The circular Motion of the Balloon was communicated to the Loop
in the Middle of one Side of the Lath

or

or Reel, round which from End to End the Twine was wrapped, and by which it hung on his Finger, and preſſed it to a Degree of Pain. *(a)*

The Work was again ſuſpended. *The Employment again ſuſpended.*

He coud not long withſtand the Temptation of indulging his Eye with a View of the glorious and enchanting Proſpect.

42. But the Beautiful among the Objects below was ſtill more attractive than the Sublime among thoſe around. *The Beautiful preferred to the Sublime, in Proſpects.*

On looking down South by Weſt, the Balloon often turning gently to the right and left, and giving the Aironaut an Opportunity of enjoying the circular View without a Change of Attitude; innumerable Rays of Light darted on the Eye as it glanced along the

---

(a) The Loop ſhoud have been furniſhed with a SWIVEL: or the Lath or Reel ſhoud have been a Kind of Pulley, a Foot in Diameter, and two Inches wide. The Hook of which having alſo a Swivel might have been held in the Hand: and thus the Twine woud have run off in a ſhort Time with the greateſt Readineſs; the Swivel conforming to the circular Motion of the Balloon. *The Defect of the Reel remedied.*

the Ground: which, tho' of a gay green Colour, appeared like an inverted Firmament glittering with Stars of the firſt Magnitude.

Inverted Firmament what.

43. This ſplendid Appearance was owing to the Rays of the Sun reflected from certain Pits or Ponds of Water, of which there is one at leaſt in moſt Fields or Incloſures throughout the County: but particularly in the low Grounds of Leach-Eye and Dodleſton.

The Object that next drew his Attention, *while aſcending*, was the Overley Turnpike-Road, which is remarkably wide, (reſembling the Emilian Way acroſs the Atrian Fens, between Bononia and Ferràra in Italy) raiſed over Saltney Marſh, leading to North-Wales and Holyhead: compoſed of Sea-Sand caſt up above high Water Mark. This appeared like a narrow Foot-Path well trodden, of a *white* Colour, and ſtrait as if drawn by a Line.

Broad Turnpike Road a narrow Foot Path.

44. No-

44. Nothing however raifed his Curiofity more than the Change in Colour of the River *Dee*, Avon ddû, (i.e. *Thee*) which in the Britifh Language fignifies the *black River*, from the Appearance of its Waters, when feen from an Eminence running in their deep Channel between the Mountains of Wales; but which glides by Chefter with a Silver Stream. This River, —Thanks to the cool Climate; not like the *green* Mincius of Virgil!—had now acquired the unvaried Colour of *red Lead*. Nor coud he difcover even the Appearance of Water; but merely that of a *broad red* Line, twining in Meanders infinitely more ferpentine than are expreffed in Maps.

River Dee red.

Whether the Change arofe from the Tranfparency of its Waters, when feen at the Height which was *apparently* 7 Miles, *as will be noticed hereafter*, though the Barometer made it fcarcely a Mile and Half, is uncertain. He was at firft inclined to think, that

Caufe of the Change conjectured.

the

the Rays, having suffered a double Refraction, were reflected to the Eye, from the reddish Sand which forms their Bottom, tho' at the Depth of 7 Yards at an Average, above the Causeway, or *artificial* Cascade near Chester Bridge: or possibly the Water of Rivers when seen at a certain Distance, may act as Water composing Clouds when view'd from below, at a certain Height and Angle; reflecting only the *red* Rays: the rest being refracted, or absorbed.

The Colours of Objects shone more brilliant and lively at that amazing Height, than if seen on a Level with themselves.

Nor did the Eye seem to want the Aid of Glasses: as every Thing, that coud be seen at all, was seen distinct.

The City of Chester *blue*.

45. The *Redness* of the River Dee was curiously contrasted by a Change equally novel but more pleasing, in the Colour of the City of Chester, when seen directly from above, on a Scale

Scale not larger than the Plan of it, in Burdett's Map.

The Town was entirely *blue*.

The higheſt Buildings had no apparent Height: their Summits were reduced to the common Level of the Ground. Nor was the Cathedral diſtinguiſhed; nor any Tower or Spire diſcerned.

The Whole had a beautiful and rich Look; not like a Model, but a coloured Map.

The Roofs of all the Houſes appeared, as if covered with *Lead*, in the moſt elegant Taſte.

Strangers may wiſh to be informed, that in moſt of the Northern Counties, the Buildings are covered with *blue Stones* called SLATES *(a)* found in the Mountains; inſtead of artificial *red* Tiles, as in London, and the South of England.

CHAP-

───────────

(a) SLATE (according to Cronſtedt) is the WHETSTONE *of fine Particles*, compoſed of Glimmer, Quartz; and, in ſome Species, of a martial argillaceous Earth. See " Eſſay on Mineralogy" by Mendes Da Coſta, Sect. 264.

CHAPTER VI.

BALLOON VERGING TO THE SEA.

Sympathy of the Spectators, on seeing the Aironaut verging towards the Sea.

Section 46. BEFORE a farther Description of aërial Scenes is attempted, it woud be improper not to mention a Circumstance which happened on the first Ascent of the Balloon: and too strongly called forth the tender sympathetic Feelings, by raising, in the Minds of the Spectators, *alarming Apprehensions* for the Safety of the Aironaut, on seeing the Balloon move gently towards the Sea.

They were however, in a great Measure, soon relieved from their Anxiety: for, by rising into another Current, he escaped the Danger: skirting the Coasts of the River Mersey; which coud not be seen from the Balloon at the Distance of little more than a League

League, tho' the Sun was supposed to shine the whole Time on the Water.

The upper Current was, in Fact, rendered visible to the aërial Traveller, for more than two Hours before, and at the Time of his Ascent; by lofty Clouds of the second Stratum, flying in a safe Direction.

CHAPTER VII.

Aërial Scenes continued.

Section 47. A Few Seconds of Time before the Balloon had attained its greatest Height; the Velocity of Ascent being every Instant retarded by the Escape of Gas thro' the Opening;—the *remarkable Stillness* which prevailed in so elevated a State of the Atmosphere, *apparently* many Miles above all visible Vapour, far beyond the Sight of every living Creature, and where the human Voice was no longer heard from below; the larger

ger Objects, with which the Surface of the distant Earth was covered, as Rivers Woods Inclosures, diminishing to the View, yet encreasing in their Beauty;—coud not but make a lively Impression on the Mind of the Aironaut.

The striking Contrast and Novelty of his Situation filled him with unusual and pleasing Sensations.

He had just left, for the first Time, his native Earth, where he had continued for a while the central Object to some *thousand* Spectators; whose Eyes, he knew, were still turned towards him; that he was still the Subject of their Conversation: yet no human Figure met his Sight; no human Sound vibrated on his Ear.

An universal Silence reigned! an empyrèan Calm! unknown to Mortals *upon Earth*.

The Sky was painted with a purer, and more transparent Azure. The Sun shone hot, and with a brighter Lustre

Luftre. His Beams were *white* and sparkling: not surrounded with Haze or Vapour: but too fierce for the human Eye to look upon a second Time with Pleasure. *(a)*

48. A Chearful Serenity filled the Breast of the Aironaut. [Objects which filled the Mind of the Aironaut with Wonder and Delight.]

In an erect Posture, and with the utmost

(a) To know whether the Air is hazy, tho' the Sun continues shining. [Method of discovering Haze round the Sun, in bright Weather.]

The Method taken for that Purpose was by placing the Hand so as to cover his Disk or Body, and then observe the Glory blazing round him; which may, in general, be seen to issue in great Abundance, in Rays of a *golden Colour*: occasioned by a Haziness or Vapour which pervades the *lower* Regions of the Air, most frequently in the hottest and calmest Weather, and in the hottest Climates. The Accumulation of these Vapours, before they are formed into Clouds, are often so great as to intercept the Sun's Rays, or dye them the Colour of Blood: an Appearance frequent in Virginia, and also throughout the torrid Zone.

In the *Campania* of Rome, for Instance, the Italians have a peculiar Name for such Kind of Weather, when the Sun is neither *visible nor invisible*: Il Sole si vede, e' non si vede.

By Degrees the Hand is to be removed so as just to have a Glance of the Sun's Limb. And it frequently happens that the Air is exceedingly hazy; tho' not a Cloud appears above the Horizon.

utmoſt Compoſure he gazed around: reflecting with Wonder and Delight on a Situation, where the BEAUTIFUL and SUBLIME were ſeen united, in a Manner perfectly novel and engaging.

Novel Situation illuſtrated by a familiar Compariſon.

If it be allowed, for the Sake of Illuſtration, to compare *great* Things with *ſmall*; he found himſelf ſuſpended in the central Concave of an unmeaſurable Crater Bowl or Baſon; and conſiderably above the Rim or Margin, ſo as to peep fairly over it: for by looking *ſtraight before him*, while the Balloon continued gently turning on its vertical Axis; he coud ſee quite round into the BLUE.

The Earth was the *Miniature-Picture (a)* painted on the Bottom of the Bowl, on the Inſide. The Sides of the Bowl next the Bottom were rather obſcure: as the Objects, on the Surface of the Earth not immediately under the Eye, being foreſhortened,

were

(*a*) Eſſe in IMAGINIBUS quâpropter *Cauſa* videtur *Cernendi*, neque poſſe SINE HIS Res ulla videri. Lucretius de Rerum Natura. L. 4. V. 238.

were indiftinct, either on Account of their immenfe Diftance, or by mere Accumulation of Vapours, and mixed with Haze and Cloudinefs.

From thence to the Top of the Bowl, was fantaftically grouped, fpoted, and dafh'd with Clouds denfe and luminous, in the ftrangeft and moft grotefque Forms; ftill fmaller and more numerous, as the Eye was more extended: The Rim or Margin ending, not in a fringed Border; but in a plain fmooth Line; to reprefent the amazing Diftance, at which, the upper Surfaces of *Clouds in Perfpective* loft all their rugged mountainous and fringed Shapes; and terminated even and fmooth: making a perfect horizontal Ring in the Heavens, fomewhat below the Eye of the Obferver. The whole formed a glorious *Concave:* and the Imagination was loft in the furrounding diftant Azure. *(a)*

The Comparifon carried on.

49. Con-

(a) Notwithftanding what has been faid; THIS, to the great and to the fordid Vulgar, woud ftill

Apparent Altitude of the Balloon when stationary.

49. Confidering more attentively the Dimenfions of this vaft Amphitheatre; as he long continued *apparently* in the *fame* Spot, and feemed to himfelf a mere Atom floating *invariably* in the Center of the empty Space; yet as a fole thinking Being there, whofe Mind was bent on eftimating the Extent of his View, fo accurately defined by the circular Horizon of denfe accumulated Vapour; and judging, as of other Diftances, by *the natural Eye* alone; pointing downwards on Objects which were only diftinguifhable when immediately below it, frequently no more than the Circuit

appear a folitary, helplefs, and deplorable Situation. But fuch are not captivated with the golden Lines of EPICTETUS, (Chap. 13. Line 3. fee Mrs. Carter's Tranflation.)

"ΠΑΝΤΑ ΘΕΩΝ μεςα και ΔΑΙΜΟΝΩΝ·— Βλεπων Ίον ΗΛΙΟΝ και Σεληνην, και Ἀςρα, και ΓΝΣ απολαυων και ΘΑΛΑΣΣΗΣ, 'ερημος εςιν ου μαλλον η και αβοηθητος." Nor are they PRACTICALLY influenced by the better Words of a much finer Writer : " The Earth is full," &c. &c. And " If I take the Wings of the Morning," &c. &c.

Circuit of a Mile on the Earth's Surface, the *vertical Boundary* of the profound Abyſs; all elſe being obſcured by Haze, or removed from Sight by Volumes of intervening Cloud; he coud not diveſt himſelf of the Idea, but that the *apparent* Depth below him was at leaſt *ſeven* Miles: *three* from the Earth to the upper Surface of the ſuperior Clouds, *(a)* and *four* above them. *(b)*

The *apparent* Heights proportioned to the *barometric* Height.

H 2 OBJECTION.

(a) There being, at firſt, no Clouds, as uſual, to occupy the Place of the loweſt Stratum.

(b) It has been ſaid that the *apparent* Height from the Balloon to the Ground was 7 Miles, viz. 4 to the Summit of the Clouds, and 3 below: and the *barometric* Height was about a Mile and half, viz. 2332 Yards, *a Calculation of which will be given.*

If then we divide that Height or Diſtance into 2 ſuch Parts, that the greater ſhall be to the leſs as 4 to 3; we obtain the Length of each Part; i. e. the barometric Height from the Balloon to the Summit of the Clouds, and thence to the Earth; which is done thus:

Suppoſe the whole Diſtance to be any Line, as A. B. to be divided in C. Then, as 7 is the whole Line, and 4 the greater Part; ſay, as the whole 7 is to the greater Part 4, ſo is the whole Diſtance to a fourth Term proportional, which will be equal to the greater Diſtance ſought:

Whole Diſtance in Yards. Greater Diſtance in Yards.
Thus 7, : 4 :: 2332 : 1332$\frac{4}{7}$ Anſ.
                     4
                   ─────
                   7)9328
2332 the whole,   1332$\frac{4}{7}$
1332$\frac{4}{7}$ being the greater Diſtance found; take the greater

Note. *The Line A. B. here ſelected is the* famous Meaſure *of (half) a* MATHEMATICAL RHinland *and* Roman FOOT, *according to Snellius. (See* Geographia Generalis *of Varenius, publiſhed by* Newton. Lib. 1. Cap. 2. De variis Menſuris.*)*

OBJECTION REMOVED.

Improbability of a concave Appearance of the Clouds and Earth, lessened, by a familiar Illustration.

50. Some may find a Difficulty in conceiving, how the whole Prospect of Clouds and Earth together coud put on a *concave* Appearance: both of which were in Reality *convex*, with Respect to the Situation of the Observer in the Car.

A familiar Illustration may help to remove the Objection.

Imagine a Person placed in the Center of a Plain, or Carpet; extended every Way beyond the Reach of the Eye. If in that Situation he was gradually elevated; the *distant* Parts of the Carpet woud *seem* to rise with him: and those Figures of the Pattern woud alone be distinguished, that lay immediately below the Eye: the more remote becoming dim and faint. The whole woud put on the Form of a

from the whole, and then will remain the lesser Distance wanted, viz. $999\frac{3}{7}$: the $1332\frac{4}{7}$ = the greater Distance, and $999\frac{3}{7}$ = the lesser Distance: and adding the Fractions $\frac{4}{7} \frac{3}{7} = 1$ to the 999; we have 1332 Yards for the greater Distance, or Height of the Balloon above the Summit of the superior Clouds: and 1000 Yards for the less Distance, or Height from the Earth to the Summit of the superior Clouds.

a concave Bowl; as foon as he had rifen to fo great a Height, as plainly to perceive the Figures of the furrounding Pattern more and more foreshortened, in Proportion to their Diftance from the Center of the Carpet.

CHAPTER VIII.

Section 51. THE Perfpective of the Clouds was entirely new; and remarkable both for Beauty and Grandeur.

The loweft Bed of Vapour that *firft* put on the Appearance of Cloud was of *a pure white*; in detached Fleeces; encreafing as they rofe. They prefently coalefced, and were aggrandized into A SEA *of Cotton*, but more *white*; and *dazling*: tufted here and there by the light Play of Air, and gentle Breezes in every Direction: but where undifturbed, the Whole became an
extended

extended Firmament or *white* Floor of thin Cloud, thro' whose Intervals the Sun must shine with fiercer Gleam. The upper Surface was quite even: not blended with the Air above, but defined and separated with the utmost Exactness; being condensed by the Coolness, and checked in their Ascent, by the Levity of the superior Regions.

Thro' this *white* Floor uprose in splendid Majesty and awful Grandeur, at great and unequal Distances, a vast Assemblage of *Thunder-Clouds*: each Congeries consisting of whole Acres in the densest Form.

52. Their conglomerate and fringed Tops rising, at different Distances, in circular Order, one above the other, to the Number of *thirty*: till they became imperceptible from their remote Situation: the Eye commanding an Extent above them of 77 Miles. *(a)*

Circular Boundary of the *celestial* Prospect from the Balloon *above* the Clouds.

Their

(a) P R O B L E M.

To find the circular Boundary of the *celestial* Prospect over the Tops of the superior Clouds, from the Balloon at the Height of near a Mile and half above the Surface of the Earth, viz. 2332 Yards. The Height from the Earth to the upper

Their Form was, as if Pieces of Ordnance were difcharged perpendicularly upwards into the Air: and that the Smoke had confolidated, at the Inftant of Explofion, into Maffes of Snow or Hail: had penetrated thro' the upper Surface or *white* Floor of common Clouds, and there remained vifible, and at Reft.

Some indeed had not wholly loft their Motion: continuing ftill to be lifted up. Others ponderous and fleepy, nodded, by mere Weight, their monftrous Heads. It feemed as if they had perfifted in mounting upwards, till they coud rife no higher: their lower Parts preffing perpendicularly

against

Surface or Floor of Clouds being 1000 Yards; and the Height above the Floor to the Balloon being 1332 Yards.
On the Curvature of the Earth and Clouds, and Elevation of the Eye above their circular Horizon.
Rule. To the Earth's Diameter, equal to 7940 geographical Miles, add *the Height* of the Eye above its Surface: multiply the Sum by that Height: then the fquare Root of the Product gives the Diftance at which an Object on the Surface of the Earth can be feen by an Eye fo elevated. Note the Diameter of the Earth, in Feet, is 41798117, according to Newton. (See Practical Navigator, by J. Moore, 7th Ed. Page 251.)

F I R S T.

Double 1000 Yards, the Height from the Earth to the Clouds for an Addition to the Diameter of the Earth, whofe

against the upper, which gradually swelled them out on *all Sides*. By partial and temporary Movements of the

Surface is now considered, as extended to the concentric Floor of Cloud.

```
        1000
        1000
        ————
        2000
```

SECOND.

```
13932702(½) Diameter of the Earth in Yards.
     2000   Addition to the Diameter.
——————
13934702   Sum, to which add
     1332  the Height of the Eye or of the
——————    Balloon above the Floor of Cloud.
13936034   Sum, which multiply into
     1332  the Height of the Eye above the
                Floor.
——————
 27872068
 41808102
 41808102
 13936034
——————
```

Extract the Square Root.

```
 . . . . .   1760) Yards in a Mile.
18562797288        (13624 5(77 Miles.
  1                 12320
 ——                ———————
23) 85              13045
    69              12320
   ———             ———————
266) 1662    Yards 440) 725( 1 Quarter of a Mile.
     1596               440
    ————               ————
2722) 6679              285 Yards.
      5444
      ————         Ans. 77 Miles, 1 Qu. 285 Yards.
27244) 123572
       108976
      ————————
272485) 1459688
        1362425
       ————————
           97263
```

Circular Boundary of the *terrestrial* Prospect from the Balloon on a *clear Day*.

PROBLEM.

To find the circular Boundary of the *terrestrial* Prospect, on

the Air, some broad *unwieldy* Caps lost the *vertical* Direction of their Columns. The Columns likewise underwent a similar and gradual Change: rolling from their Pedestals or spiral Bases; and, at Times, assuming EVERY ORGANIZED SHAPE that Fancy coud suggest.

53. The imperceptibly slow yet perpetual Changes they underwent, strongly called to Remembrance, the

Opinion of Philosophers.

I Opinion

a clear Day, from the Balloon at the Height of near a Mile and half, viz. 2332 Yards: the Earth's Diameter being
```
          equal to 13932705⅔ Yards,
              add     2332  the Height of the Eye or
                            Balloon.
                  ─────────
                  13935037  the Sum, multiply into
                      2332  the Height of the Eye, &c.
                  ─────────
                  27870074
                  41805111
                  41805111
                  27870074
                  ─────────
Extract the   .  .  .  .  .     1760) Yards in a Mile.
square Root   32496506284     (180267(102,
                    1          1760 say 102½ Miles. Ans.
                 ─────          ────
              28)224            4267
                 224            3520
                 ───            ────
              3602) 9650          747 Yards, Remainder.
                    7204
                    ────
              36046)244662
                    216276
                    ──────
             360527) 2838684
                     2523689
                     ───────
                      314995 Remainder.
```

Opinion of the great Berkeley, *(a)* as well as of the ancient Philosophers, that AIR GIVES FORM TO THINGS: scarcely a Breath of which seemed, however, to disturb their general Order.

The Constitution of these enormous Masses was such as to reflect *some* of the Sun's Rays, and to transmit *others* in a Variety of Colouring.

The Colours of the Thunder Clouds.

54. The Parts next the Sun were of a *snowy* Whiteness. Then of a *bright luminous Yellow* melting into a *dusky Sulphur*: afterwards of a *Purple*. The Rays being now shorn; a Degree of Opacity and Transmission took Place throu' half the Substance of the Cloud, which seemed of a *transparent Blue* like the *Onyx*.

Delightful Tints visible only from the Balloon.

55. These *delightful Tints* must be ever eclipsed to a Spectator on the Surface of the Earth, looking upwards throu' the gross Atmosphere that surrounds it; but highly *interesting* to one who

is

(a) See his " Minute Philosopher."

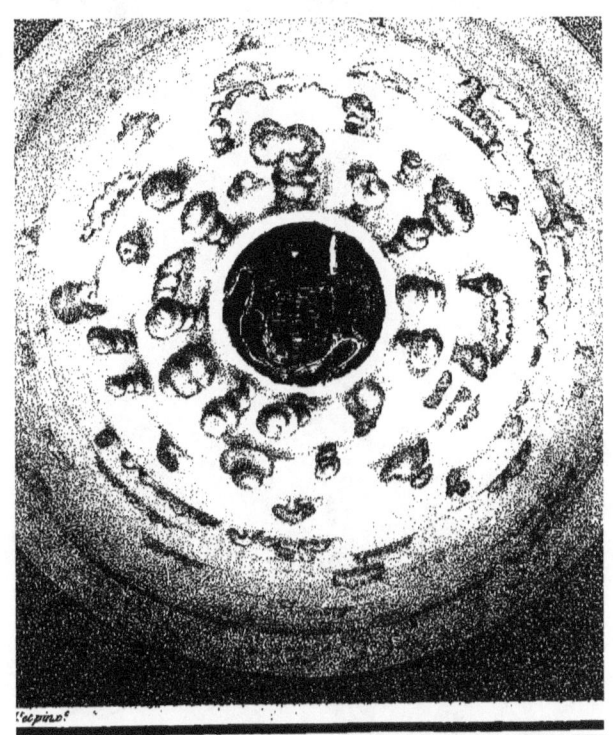

A VIEW from the **BALLOON** *at its* **GREATEST** *elevation see Page* IIII. *a.*

Publish'd May 1.ˢᵗ 1786, by T. Baldwin Chester.

is suspended in a rarified and unencumbered Medium of the etherial Regions, where the Eye darts without Resistance above Clouds, and all visible Vapour.

Note: the Print, representing a circular View from the Balloon at its greatest Elevation, is taken from a Scene described in the above Chapter.

CHAPTER IX.

OTHER AERIAL SCENES DESCRIBED.

Section 56. DURING the Time that the Balloon from being stationary at $23\frac{1}{4}$ (corresponding to the Height of about a Mile and a half) began to *decline*, which it must have done with a brisk Motion, imperceptible to the Aironaut at the Time, tho' since recognized, on Account of the great Opening at the Bottom; he traced its *Shadow* over

Balloon Shadow traced on the Clouds.

the Tops of Volumes of Clouds below. It was at firſt ſmall: in Size and Shape like an Egg: but ſoon encreaſed to the Magnitude of the Sun's Diſk; and woud have made a ſolar Eclipſe to a Spectator looking from the Cloud: ſtill growing larger, as the Balloon deſcended, or Clouds aroſe. But his Attention was preſently called to another equally novel, but more captivating Appearance; that of an *Iris* encircling the whole *Shadow*, at ſome Diſtance round it. The Colours were remarkably brilliant.

This *celeſtial Phantom* attended the Aironaut for a few Minutes: conforming, as a Veſſel at Sea, to the Change of *Surface*; now plainly viſible, now indiſtinct and diſappearing; as it paſſed *throu'* the *luminous* or *ſhadowy Wave* of Clouds *apparently* at Reſt.

The Iris, a Frame to the pictured Land, vaniſhes.

57. The Clouds, in which this Phenomenon continued, were of the ſuperior or ſecond Stratum in Height, as in fair

fair Weather; rare; of a transparent *Blue* and purest *White*, alternate. At the End of four Minutes they dispersed, so as to admit an unexpected Sight of the pictured Land thro' THEM, and thro' the Place of *the Balloon-Shadow*; whose Form first vanishing, *the Iris* remained, for a few Seconds, complete, and in resplendent Beauty.

58. *I'rides*, of the same Kind, tho' of less vivid Colours, are seen round the Moon, in a mild Evening; as thin light Clouds move slowly under it. (*a*)

59. The Sun shone brighter and fiercer, when the Balloon was at its greatest Height; the *Heat* piercing throu' his Cloths, (which were of a *dark* Colour;) while the Aironaut *stood* with his Face from the Light.

The Mouth remaining open, it continued

<small>Sun hottest when the Balloon was stationary.</small>

<small>Lunardi's Flag thrown out, at the Height of a Mile.</small>

(*a*) Ullòa in his Voyage to South-America relates, that in passing over the DESERTS, I'rides are frequently seen by Travellers round *their own Heads* as the Center of the *Iris*; and visible only to themselves. But what Analogy the *Balloon Iris* bears to them, Time and future Experiments may discover. See his "Voyage to South America, Vol. 1. Pa. 442."

tinued to descend, as appeared by the Barometer which had risen nearly to 24 Inches: at which Instant Mr. Lunardi's *coloured* Flag was thrown out, for the Information of a Friend; and that Spectators below might judge what was nearly the perpendicular Height of a Mile in the Air, according to Halley's Table.

The Flag was seen to descend for 3 Minutes.

60. The Flag was seen by the Aironaut to descend for three Minutes: at which Time it became invisible. It fell, *not* perpendicularly; but in large Spirals, and by Jerks; darting first on one Side, then on the other. The Resistance of the Air made it act as a Parashute. The Flag was instantly pursued, and taken up in a Field one Mile distant from Chester. The Descent of the Balloon must have been retarded, being four Pounds and a half lighter.

The Dove turned out.

61. The Pigeon was then taken out of the Basket of Matting: Thermometer 54; Barometer $25\frac{1}{10}$. It trembled

bled much. Being turned loose, it looked frequently up at the Car; but flew downwards in cylindrical Gyrations eight or ten Yards in Diameter, according to the Turn of its Head to the right, which seemed to rest in an oblique Attitude: the Wings and Tail continuing extended as much as possible, but without Motion, during its Descent. The Bird was out of Sight in a few Minutes: but continued, as *the Owner* observed, full half an Hour, in the Air.

CHAPTER X.

Section 62. A T 10 Minutes and a half past II. o'Clock, the fourth or last Cannon, a Sixpounder (to announce, by preconcerted Agreement, that the Balloon began to be invisible to Spectators in the Castle-Yard, Chester) was distinctly

_{4th Cannon heard,}

tinctly heard by the Aironaut; but had no Effect on the Balloon: did not agitate it in the leaft: the contrary of which was expected.

For the fame Cannon, difcharged the third Time at the Diftance of 30 Yards from the Balloon, when it had rifen a few Feet from the Ground; affected it fo ftrongly, that the Aironaut was THEN ONLY obliged to keep himfelf upright, by holding the Cords with his Hands.

Balloon firft invifible to the Inhabitants of Chefter.

63. At 17 Minutes paft II. was heard the Sound of a Number of Voices, which it was then imagined came from Chefter, as the farewel Salute after the laft Cannon: but it was afterwards known that the Balloon did not become wholly invifible, till that Shout.

Diftance of the Balloon calculated.

64. From an Obfervation made by a Spectator in the Caftle-Yard, juft half an Hour intervened between the Difcharge of the third, and of the laft Cannon; as therefore the Report was half

DECEPTION OF THE SIGHT.

half a Minute, or 30 Seconds *(a)* longer in reaching the Balloon; the Diftance of the Balloon at the Time of the Report was *nearly* fix Miles and a half.

64. The fingle thin white Cloud of the firft or loweft Order in Height that rendered Chefter invifible to the Aironaut, was obferved feveral Minutes before, *apparently* to pafs under the Balloon, retire from it, to approach, and expected to invelope, the *blue* City of Chefter: which for a long Time had been kept in View, and feen *obliquely,* under the *common* Perfpective, with a fmall Degree of Elevation above the Level of the Ground: fuggefting to his Mind the curious and complete Model of Paris, exhibited fome

<small>Chefter feen as a *fmall* Model.</small>

K

(a) As Sound travels - - - - - 1142 Feet in a Second, it muft have moved in - - - 30 Seconds

Feet in a Yard - - 3)34260=Feet
Yards in a Mile 1760)11420(6 Miles
 10560

Yards in a Quarter of a Mile 440)860(1 Quarter
 440

Anfwer 6 Miles, 1 Quarter, and 420 Yards.

some Years ago *on a small Table*, in many Towns of Europe.

The Sight doubly deceived in the Distance.
The Cloud appeared, four Miles Distance at least from the Aironaut; below; and as if touching the City. The contrary Supposition, it seems, took Place, among the Inhabitants there: who thought, a Cloud, a Mile above them, had surrounded and inveloped the Balloon.

Condiments tasted as usual.
65. The Pepper Salt and Ginger were tasted, and found to retain their usual Pungency: contrary to what Travellers have reported to happen on the Peak of Teneriffe.

Silk electric.
The small Hank of yellow raw Silk tyed to the upper Hoop, and hanging down from it, appeared *rough*, as if electric: and, tho' drawn thro' the Hand, continued *furred* as before.

White Flag wholly hung out from the Car.
66. It was now thought a proper Time to finish the original Work of unwinding the remaining Part of the half Mile of Twine: which proved equally tedious, as at the first; and took

took up a considerable Time. When completed, the *white* Flag was extended exactly half a Mile from the Car.

67. Perceiving that the Balloon was descending very *briskly*, by the Appearance of Cattle in the Corner of a Field; first, *one* of the two solid Weights was cast down: then the other. *Cattle discovered from the Balloon. Ballast thrown out,*

A Return of Sound to the Balloon, from the lighter which weighed five Pounds, was heard in 130 Countings of a Watch, which made 120 of the same full Beats in a Minute. *Time in falling estimated.*

Before the Weight became invisible; it *appeared* to move a good Deal out of the Perpendicular: owing either to an under Current; or to a Deception of Sight, respecting the horizontal Motion of the Balloon in a different Direction, during the Descent of the Stone.

The other muſt have fallen in ſoft Graſs, or otherwiſe: as it was not heard.

CHAPTER XI.

Section 68. AT 28 Minutes paſt II. the ſolid Weights before mentioned were thrown out.

At 29 Minutes the Barometer had fallen to 25 Inches.

Balloon reaſcending. A Handful of Feathers were ſent adrift, which fell quick: demonſtrating *likewiſe* the Aſcent of the Balloon, a ſecond Time: but, tho' 12 Pounds lighter, it did not ſeem to regain its original Height: judging MERELY from this Circumſtance, that no more Gaſs eſcaped *viſibly* from the Mouth.

Apparent Size and Situation of the white Flag. 69. It is ſomewhat remarkable, that, on repeated Enquiries from unprejudiced Perſons, the *white* Flag, when ſuſpended from the Car above 440 Yards, appeared 4 Yards long: and when

when at the end of the *half Mile* Twine, feemed about 8 Yards long, to Spectators from below, in different Places: that fometimes it appeared before, and fometimes behind the Balloon: while to the Obferver in the Car, it feemed regularly to follow the Balloon: unlefs when a *new* Motion was impreffed upon the latter: at which Time the *white* Flag was fituated almoft under the Car: or when the Balloon changed its Direction; the Flag being *then* not always *difcoverable*.

When feen *edgewife* or *forefhortened*; it woud *appear* to be *nearer* the Car than it really was.

70. As there was a Peculiarity attending the Situation of the *half Mile* Flag, which may prove of fingular Ufe in Airoftation; it ought not to be paffed over in Silence.

Effect of the white Flag on the Balloon.

The half Mile Flag hanging loofely from the Car; not perpendicularly under, but following it, frequently at

an

an Angle of about 45 Degrees; shews that the Flag met a Resistance from the Air, unfelt by the Balloon: which out strip'd it, in Proportion to the *greater* Surface which the Balloon exposed to the Wind.

Taking also into the Account, that the Balloon remained in Equilibrio; while the Flag was subject to the Force of Gravity: which Force was restrained from Exertion, otherwise than as a *Vis Inertiæ*, to keep it always in a perpendicular Situation.

The Resistance of the Air, acting in an horizontal Direction against the *Vis Inertiæ* of the Flag, must have a Tendency to drive it back: which being ineffectual; the Flag must consequently *rise*; and in rising *will retard the Balloon.*

A Power may therefore be communicated to a Balloon, in the Direction of the Wind, which shall *retard* its Progress throu' the Air: a Subject which

which seems capable of farther Prosecution.

CHAPTER XII.

Section 71. FROM 28 Minutes after II, till the Balloon had passed over the *Forest* of DELAMERE, and the steep Crag of HELSBYE-HILL; thin light semi-transparent Vapours, which seemed to be collecting at a *vast Depth below*; moving slowly in all Directions; rising to great Heights, falling, melting away, and again condensing;—(the Land, one while covered with a WHITE *Veil*; then *caught* thro' Openings for a few Seconds; the Objects appearing more distinct and *coloured,* from being seen in detached Groupes and single *Pictures framed* and *enshrined* in fleecy VAPOUR; *now again* discovered by a Glance of the Eye, and *then* repeatedly escaping from the

Beautiful Effects of the white Vapour on the Prospects below.

the Sight;)—WONDERFULLY heightened the Grandeur, Gaiety and *inimitable* Beauty of the *ever varying* Prospects.

An Illustration taken from Scenes abroad.

72. Appearances of a similar Kind are frequent in the *noble and venerable* Structures appropriated for divine Worship *abroad:* whose Walls are decorated with the *finest Paintings*; the Subjects solemn and *engaging*; suited to inspire a *chearful Devotion.*

While the inferior Clerics perfume the Garments of the *Priests* officiating and offering Incense before the *high Altar*; which is ornamented with *full-Length Portraits* in the richest Drapery, of Persons whether male or female, reputed of sound Morals and exemplary Piety; accompanied by Guardian Saints and happy Angels;—Columns of *white* Smoke, wafted from *Silver* Censers, rise to a certain Height in slow *majestic* Movement, before the Eyes of the *kneeling* Suppliants, who are *instantly shut out* from the *enchanting* View;

View; till the Clouds difperfing, fhew by *Intervals*, a Glympfe of the *celeftial* Profpect, and of the *higher* Orders of Beings, who *look down* with *Complacency* upon them; and feem *actually* DESCENDING throu' Openings of the Clouds which *appear* at Reft.

CHAPTER XIII.

Section 73. AT 33 Minutes after II, the Balloon-Shadow was *again* the Center of a brilliant *Iris*, painted at fome Diftance round it on Clouds below. 2d Balloon-Iris.

74. One of the Pint-Bottles for light Air was prepared (as in Article 14, of Section 12;) and dropped from the Car. Bottle filled with *light* Air.

The *Water* it contained was poured down

down, to obferve the Effects of *Air* and *Light* on the Drops.

The Air did *not* at that Height oppofe a Refiftance fufficient to break the Stream into *fmall* Drops. Nor did they feem to coalefce: remaining, while they continued in Sight, of the fame Size; fome very large, others lefs fo; and at the fame *relative* Diftance, as when they firft left the Bottle.

The Colours feemed *ftronger* than ufual.

It may be *here* obferved that none of the Bottles were returned; tho' found, and a Reward promifed.

The Country People, as foon as they faw a Bottle; imagining it muft contain fome Liquor, immediately contrived to open it: by which Procedure, the Intention of the Experiment was fruftrated.

The Bottles, which are *dangerous* Companions even without Liquor, fhoud,

fhoud, notwithftanding, be left in the Car: at leaft till the Time of *landing* the Balloon.

75. While the Balloon was *firft* rifing; a gentle Motion of the lower Current of Air carried it immediately towards the Sea. (Section 46.) *Burton and Flint feen at the firft rifing.*

At which Time, the Aironaut by a *Glance* difcovered the Mouth of the River Dee, four and five Miles wide, *yawning before him:* the Profpect extending to the Sea, as far as the *Smoke* from the Lead-Works near a Place called Flint on the Welch Coaft; and to Burton-Head on the Wirral Side; diftant ten Miles from Chefter.

He has fince been informed; that the Balloon feemed to REST, for a few Minutes, in the Air: and then *return flowly* over Chefter.

It is therefore more than probable, that as the Balloon continued to afcend; it was *becalmed* in a *quiefcent Stratum* or Bed of the Atmofphere, *Balloon in a quiefcent Bed of Air.* which

which existed for a certain Depth or Thickness, between the lower and upper Current: and that the Direction of the Balloon was changed; the Instant it arrived within the Influence of the *upper* Current.

Of rowing the Balloon to any Point of the Compass.

Consequently, with a proper Apparatus to ascend and descend *at Will*, without Loss of Gass or Ballast; the Balloon woud have remained suspended *invariably* at the same Height, and *vertically* over the same Spot of Earth: or, with propulsive Machinery; might, on the same Level, have been *rowed* to any Point of the Compass.

The Balloon, influenced on its Approach towards Water.

76. In passing *only* ACROSS Trafford Meadows, three Miles from Chester; the Balloon lost its usual progressive Motion over the Country: for more than a Quarter of an Hour, following the Course of the River Goway to the West North-West, and towards the Sea, as at Chester: turning gently backwards and forwards round its own Axis,

Axis, near the Villages of Great and Little Barrow: and making Curves over the Meadows, whose Breadth at those Places was about a Mile.

The Balloon then returned into its former Direction: inclining, *again*, towards a Brook and Meadow near Alvanley: passed Eastward a little to the left of Manley *(white)* Mill: crossed the Forest of Delamere, and Crag of Helsbye, (about twice the Height of Shooter's Hill, near London;) whose lofty Summit was *apparently* reduced to a common Level with the Valley made by the River Wever, and with the adjacent Sea Marsh. Nor coud it have been distinguished by a Stranger, as an *Eminence*. Its Progress marked.

Indeed, the Wood near Kingsley, which grows on a sloping Ground, skirting the Hill, and *from* the Sun, put on a *dusky* Hue; and the Tops of the Trees a *darker Green:* this Difference of *Colour*, conveyed the *faint Resemblance* of a rising SLOPE. A Hills and Vallies on a Level.

real

real Knowledge of the Country probably contributed to aid the Imagination in this Diſtinction.

Note: the Print repreſenting a View of the Balloon over *Helſbye Crag*, refers to a Scene in the above Chapter.

CHAPTER XIV.

<small>39 Minutes paſt II, Frodſham Town and Bridge ſeen.</small>

Section 77. AT 39 Minutes after II, Thermometer 60, Barometer $23\frac{3}{4}$, correſponding to the Height of a little more than a Mile (*a*), *the Vapours diſperſing*, diſcovered the Town of Frodſham, and Bridge over the Wever diſtant from the Town one Mile: the Balloon ſtill continuing at a vaſt Height; having riſen imperceptibly from the Time that the Ballaſt was thrown down.

From a Converſation held the next Morning at Frodſham, with ſome intelligent Perſons who had deſcried

(*a*) Equal to 2085 Yards; or 1 Mile, 325 Yards.

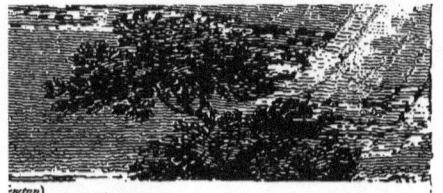

The BALLOON *over* HELS

Published

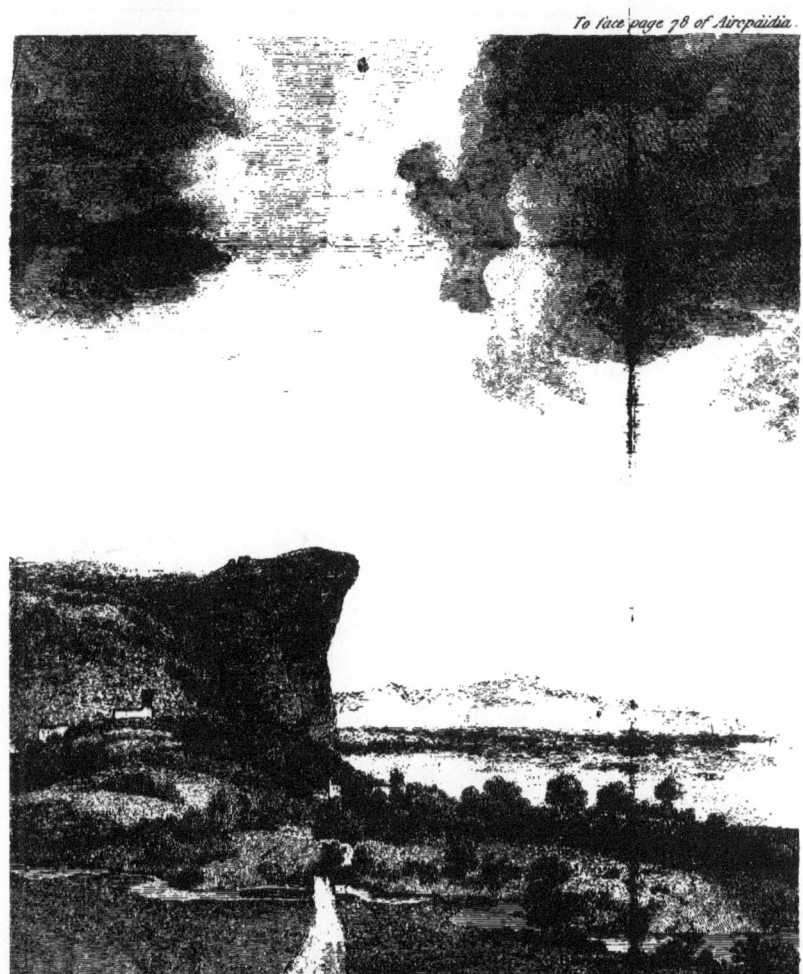

The BALLOON over HELSBYE HILL in CHESHIRE see page IIII b.

Published May 1, 1786, by T. Baldwin Chester.

cried it gliding gently throu' the Air; the Balloon appeared fo extremely *minùte*, that it was thought impoffible to be the ONE expected the fame Day to rife at Chefter with an Aironaut.

To ufe their own Expreffion, " *it coud not have been larger than a Bladder, if they had feen it on the Ground.*" The fame Perfons obferved the *white* Flag, like a *Feather* about 8 Yards Diftance from the Balloon.

<small>Half Mile *white* Flag like a Feather.</small>

A fecond Air Bottle was thrown down.

78. The Town of Kingfley being to the Eaft; Frodfham-Bridge half a Mile to the Weft; the Conflux of the Rivers Wever, and the *wide* Merfey falling into the Sea one Mile farther Weftward; the Balloon proceeding in its ufual Courfe over the Country in the *upper* Current; began to be *impeded*, on its vertical Approach ACROSS the Meadows to the Wever: was actually ftopped; and being *entangled* by the

<small>Courfe of the Balloon traced to fhew the Manner in which it was affected by the *Water*.</small>

the *River*, evidently changed its former Direction: imitating, if possible, *its* Meanders; or at least making Gyrations in Circles of different Diameters, at the same Time turning different Ways round its Axis: describing Curves, something similar to that of the Moon round the Earth in her Orbit; or of Saturn, Jupiter, and Mars, as those *Curves* are delineated in the *Prints* of Long's Astronomy: *(a)* the Course of the River being its *changeable* Center.

79. It is to be observed, that if the Balloon had continued to pursue its *former* Course; no Danger was to be apprehended of its falling on the Sea, or on the broad Branch of the River Mersey towards Warrington.

On the contrary, it must have gone into the Heart of the adjoining County, and passed near Manchester.

It is likewise worthy of remark; that unless a Fragment of light Vapour

(a) Long's Astronomy. Pages 227, 229.

pour intervened for a few Seconds; the Country immediately below the Obferver was *continually* illuminated by the Sun's Rays: tho' none but the larger Objects were diftinguifhable at the Bottom of the profound Abyfs, *more* than two Miles in Diameter at one View: that being the utmoft Boundary of the circular Profpect below.

80. The *Sea* tho' known to be *near* by the Dafhing of its Waves upon the Shore, which were plainly heard, was then totally eclipfed: as if by Haze or Vapour, which began to be accumulated only at a certain Height *below* the Balloon; yet in fuch a Manner as *not* to prevent the folar Rays from penetrating throu', and fhining bright upon the Water.

<small>Circularity of Profpect below, bounded by *Vapour*.</small>

81. There was now fufficient Leifure to trace the incredible Variety of moft beautiful *Curves*, into which the Stream had worked the Bed of the River Wever in a Courfe of *Time*, and in the

M   Compafs

Compass of a few Miles: an Appearance which *demonstrates* the Incorrectness of MAPS.

Some *actual* Clouds presented themselves in detached Groupes over the Land; and the *Land* itself *shone* plainer throu' the Intervals, than in Places near which *no* Clouds appeared.

82. On reconnoitring the scattered Town of Frodsham, which like Chester was of a *light* BLUE; the Balloon moving *by Intervals* round its Axis, the Prospect seemed to *open* on a *sudden*; and the Aironaut coud discover the Town of Warrington: the Plan of which was small, neat, but of a *darker Blue*, inclining to *Grey*: the Slates *(a)* there used being almost peculiar to the County of Lancaster.

Sight of Warrington.

83. From this *Enlargement* of the Prospect over Land, he imagined that the Balloon was either *gently* descending;

(a) Also called the *Horsham Stone*, from a Place so named, in Surrey, where great Quantities are found.

ing; or that it appeared throu' the *clear* Intervals of *actual* Clouds *below* him.

84. He had Time however to make the following Remarks. Cattle, if grazing in the Meadows, were not distinguishable; or at least were not distinguished. It was in vain to look for Sheaves of Corn, or Hattocks on the Ground: possibly from a Sameness of *Colour* like the growing *Stalks*, and *Field*: or *protruding* but a small Degree of ELEVATION; tho' the *Shadow* even at *twelve o'Clock (a)* was something longer.

(a) P R O B L E M.
To find the *Length* of the *Shadow* from a Person of *middle* Stature, (five Feet and a half High) viz. at XII o'Clock, on the 8th Day of September, 1785, at Chester, whose North Latitude, is 53° 12′; (and 3° 11′ West Longitude from London.)
F I R S T,
To find the Sun's Altitude at XII.
From 90°. 00′ Subtract
The Latitude 53. 12

The Remain. 36. 48 is the Complement of Latitude, to which add (from the Tables)
Sun's N. Decl. 5. 29

The Remain. 42. 17 is the Sun's Altitude (viz. at XII.)
S E C O N D,
For the Shadow say,
As the Sine of the Sun's Altitude, 42° 17′
To the Person's Height, viz. 66 Inches,
So is the Co-Sine of the Sun's Altitude,
To the Length of the Shadow.
For the Sine of the Sun's Altitude 42° 17′ in the Table

longer than the *perpendicular* Height of EACH Object. *(b)* Noises of Carriages along the great Turnpike-Road; especially Waggons and Carts HEAVILY laden; (the Gratings of whose *Wheels* against the *Stones* seemed uncommonly *harsh*;) were discriminately heard, tho' not *discoverable* by the Eye. Numbers of human Voices were almost CONTINUALLY huzzaeing:

<small>Pleasurable Circumstance peculiar to the Balloon.</small>

of artificial Sines, is the Logarithm 9.82788, which, subtracted from the arithmetic Complement, viz. 9.99999 (supposing the last Figure a 10) becomes, - - - - .17212
Then for the Person's Height, viz. 66 Inches: in the Table of Logarithms is the corresponding Number, - - - - - - - - - - - 1.81254
And for the Co-Sine (had by subtracting the Altitude 42.17 from 90.00) viz. 47.43: among the artificial Sines is the Logarithm, - - - - - 9.86913

The above Sums added, are - - - - - - 11.86079 which logarithmic Number (deducting the *Initial* 1 as useless) viz. 1.86079, in the Table of Logarithms, corresponds to 72.57, equal to 72 Inches, for the Length of the Shadow at XII.
  Reducing then the Numbers 66 and 72, to the lowest Denomination, thus $6)\frac{66}{72}=\frac{11}{12}$ the Proportion which the *Length* of the *Shadow* bears to the *Height* of the *Object* is thereby obtained: that is.
  (b) If the *Length* of the Shadow be divided into 12 Parts, the Height of the Object would be 11 of those Parts.
          See Moore's Practical Navigator.

PROBLEM.

An EASY Way to find the Proportion which the *Length* of the Shadow bears to the *Height* of an Object is, AT ANY TIME WHEN THE SUN SHINES, to fix a Plummet Line and FRAME *upright* in the Ground; measure the *Length* of its *Shadow*, and compare *it* with the *Height* of the FRAME.

ing: except while STATIONARY at the firſt Riſe; when ALL AROUND was wrapt in the Sublimity of SILENCE; which afforded a pleaſurable Contraſt;—diffuſing a DELICIOUS CALM.

A third Bottle of Air was thrown out.

CHAPTER XV.

Section 85. AT 4 Minutes paſt III, the Balloon remained *vertically* over the River, and over the elegant Manſion called Afton. Balloon over Afton-Houſe, at 4 Minutes paſt III, and near a Mile high.

86. A Wind was heard BELOW for a few Seconds: and the Air felt a *little cool*. Thermometer 55, or Temperate: Barometer $25\frac{1}{2}$, correſponding to the Height of near a Mile. *(a)* Wind *below*.

87. The Balloon continuing its eccentric Movements from *Side to Side* acroſs the The Balloon going to Sea, determined the Aironaut to *deſcend*, in Hopes of finding a Sea-Breeze in Time.

(a) Equal to 3 Quarters of a Mile and 121 Yards.

the Meadows; yet ſtill gliding *down* the River, in a North-Weſt by North Direction, almoſt at right Angles to that which it *before* had held; conſequently *towards* the Sea, and in a Line which continued muſt paſs thro'' the Center of the Channel: ſome Step it was neceſſary to take, and SOON. By throwing out Ballaſt, the Balloon woud inſtantly riſe: but it woud probably, as *before*, riſe into A CALM, and therefore *deſcend* nearly in the ſame Line: which woud merely *protract* the Time till the Balloon had reached the Center of the Channel: where, having no Reſource, the Ballaſt being then expended; there might be ſome Riſque in waiting for a Veſſel, tho' the Balloon woud not for SEVERAL HOURS, have loſt its *levitating* Power, ſo as to have ſunk with the Aironaut. To him however it immediately occurred, that there might be an UNDER Current of Air, as uſual in the Middle of the Day, blowing

ing from Sea to Land: and, that if the Balloon was made to descend QUICKLY into the Sea-Breeze; it might, in a few Minutes, be carried so *far* within the Country, as to be *soon beyond* the Influence of the *Sea* and *River*: and THEN, by throwing out some Pounds of Ballast, woud return into the *upper* Current, and pursue a *safe* Course towards Manchester; or even towards Prescot and Liverpool, if an easterly Wind prevailed *above*.

88. In Consequence of these Expectations; he looked downwards *towards* the Sea, *then* wholly *invisible*; tho' the Murmuring of its Waves was *more* plainly heard.

THICK SMOKES were distinguished issuing from *different* Places along the Marsh near the Coast: and *apparently* skirting the Ground, as if impelled by a *brisk* Wind from the Sea.

<small>Smoke blown to Land by a Sea-Breeze.</small>

89. No Time was to be lost.

The Balloon having reached the Cascade; and continuing to move

more

more regularly along the Courſe of the River, paſt the *Bridge*, and proceeded to *Rock-Savage*.

The Balloon ſtill going to Sea, the Mouth was opened.

90. The Neck or *Mouth* which remained ſhut, by its own Preſſure againſt the Outſide of the upper Hoop, as *it* lay over it; was inſtantly brought within the Hoop, and ſet WIDE OPEN in a perpendicular Situation.

Not more than a Couple of Minutes had elapſed before Sounds were more audible and louder.

Cattle and Corn in the Fields became viſible.

Ballaſt in Hand ready to throw out.

91. The Obſerver very deliberately ſtooping to put down his Card and Pencil; with his *left* Hand graſping the Hoop of the Car, and with his Right holding a Sand-Bag, to throw over as he approached the Earth; found that the Balloon was *influenced* by an UNDER Current blowing from the Sea: and marked his Progreſs by the half Mile WHITE Flag; whoſe Stretcher having acquired a Poſition parallel

parallel to the Plane of the Horizon, placed the Flag in an excellent Point of View: the Balloon *towing* it *apparently* with a *slow* Motion, over the distant Tops of the *dark-green* Trees.

CHAPTER XVI.

BALLOON DESCENDING.

Section 92. NO sooner had the Balloon *descended* within the Influence of the *Sea Breeze*, than it became INSTANTLY *condensed* by a certain CHILLINESS which THEN began to prevail. Air chilly.
Therm. 55;
Barom. 26½.

93. This Height has *since* been considered as the LEVEL of FLEECY VAPOUR, SCUD, or lowest Stratum of Clouds, in BRIGHT and WARM Weather.(*a*) Balloon in the under Current.

No *visible* Clouds were presented *near* the Spectator. On the contrary, they seemed to *shrink back* to the Distance of a Mile round the Eye; and then immediately

---

(*a*) i.e. When the Barometer *below* is at 30 Inches, and Thermometer *below* at 60° viz. about 1000 Yards high in *fine* Weather, and 500 in *changeable*.

immediately appear above it, the Balloon continuing to defcend. Nor did any *circular* Horizon of the Earth fhew itfelf; till the Balloon had reached below this Level: viz. Barom. 26½, Thermom. 55. i. e. Temperate.

Profpects were moft EXTENSIVE and beautiful at this Altitude: which the Barometer eftimates at full half a Mile. *(a)*

Looking again at the Barometer, fcarce a Minute afterwards; it had rifen to 27.

<small>Sudden Effect of cool moift Air on the Balloon.</small> 94. The Condenfation by Chill and Moifture, and quick Contraction of *its* Dimenfions acted like a *Charm* on the *Balloon.*

In a Moment; as if dropped from the Clouds, the SEA fuddenly prefented itfelf. *(b)* It feemed NEAR, and of a RED Colour. *Circular* Landfcapes of the *diftant* Countries filled the Eye.

Almoft

(a) Being 1083 Yards, i. e. half a Mile, and 203 Yards.

(b) It was High Water at Chefter and Frodfham-Bridge, at 38 Minutes paft I.

Almoſt the whole Extent of the Channel was a perfect Calm: and rather *dazled* the Sight. But from the Peninſula of Hale to that of Runcorn, and upwards, a *partial* BREEZE from the North-Weſt *ruffled* the Surface (which was there of a *dark* and menacing Complexion;) and ſeemed in its Courſe to have reached and *influenced* the Balloon: whoſe Deſcent proving *more* rapid than was expected; the Sand-Bag tyed up, weighing 12 Pounds, was opened, and the Sand *diſperſed*.

95. The Aironaut continuing as before to *ſtand* upright in the Car, and having reſumed his Card and Pencil; Thermometer *again* at 55°, on finding the Deſcent not *ſufficiently* retarded, wrote ſwiftly, "NO MORE REMARKS, MIND THE SHIP:" meaning the Balloon: and briſkly ſtooping for the ſecond Bag of Sand, weighing likewiſe 12 Pounds, *diſperſed* it by *Handfulls* in the ſame Manner.

Ballaſt thrown down, 12lb. and 12lb.

96. The

BALLOON MADE TO DESCEND RAPIDLY.

Defcent at firft rapid.

96. The circular Mouth of the Balloon continuing wide open, at about 18 Inches Diameter; fo much *cool* and *moift* Air rufhed in during the Defcent; that, tho' its Momentum or acquired Motion was retarded by *Difperfion* of the Ballaft, it had not yet recovered an ACTUAL LEVITY: being too near the Ground before the fecond Bag was difcharged.

Prefuming however that 24 Pounds Weight of Ballaft thrown out, was fufficient to break the Fall, tho' in a cool moift *condenfing* Atmofphere of *pure defloguifticated* Air; the Event of *landing* was *waited for*.

A depreffing Torrent of Air on the Balloon.

It has been *fince* imagined that a *heavy* DEPRESSING Torrent of *cool* Air took Place from the North-Weft at a certain Height over the Water, and *affifted* the Defcent of the Balloon.

The Balloon defcended with a rufhing Noife.

97. In order to judge with what Rapidity the Balloon defcended, when fo LOW as to be within the Influence of the *under* Current, while the

the *cool moist* Air rushed in at the Bottom, and most probably pressed out the Gass; the following Intelligence has been communicated by a Person of Veracity.

As two credible Farmers were working, with their Servants, in the HARVEST; on hearing a hollow, rushing Sound in the Air, which they took to be a *Whirl-wind*, or *distant Thunder*, and which seemed every Moment to encrease and approach them; they all retreated under a large Oak. While there, they first perceived the swift Descent of the Balloon. Two, who were afraid of Thunder, then began to take Courage, boldly exclaiming they shoud never fear Thunder again, since the *Falling* of a Balloon coud be attended with so *terrible* a Noise.

Anecdote shewing the Rapidity of Descent, at first.

CHAP-

CHAPTER XVII.

BALLOON STILL DESCENDING.

Section 98. THE Car, gliding *over* Trees in the *farther* Hedge-Row of a Grafs Field, glanced on the Ground.

Caution on Landing.

The Aironaut, being *prepared* for the Event, fupported a *Part* of the Weight of his Body by his Hands, grafping the *upper* Hoop.

The Balloon *ftooping*, and declining from the North-Weft Breeze, drew the *upper* Hoop out of the Perpendicular: by which Means, the Bottom of that Divifion of the Barometer-Frame which contained the *Tube*, preffed againft the Bottom of the Car on the Ground, was *feparated* from the remaining Half of the Frame, and fell on the *Grafs*.

The Balloon, then rifing with an elaftic *Bound*, elevated the Car a few Yards,

Yards, and descended to the Ground, but *more* gently than before: rose again; and the Aironaut perceiving that the progressive Motion of the Breeze was bringing the Balloon near a *third* Hedge; took up his Knife, (which lay by him *ready open* for Use) and *cut away* the remaining Half of the *Barometer-Frame*; threw out the *Basket with the Bottles*, and *Tunning Dish*; the *Speaking Trumpet*; the *Woollen Gloves*, the remaining half Mile of *Twine on the Reel.* (a) [More Ballast parted with, viz. seven Pounds.]

The Car *cleared* the Hedge, and *slightly* for *an Instant* touched Ground, the *third* Time.

99. During these Operations; the Aironaut had observed different Per- [Farmers offering their Assistance.]
sons

(a) Articles parted with, to check the *first* Descent at Bellair, near Frodsham: and to ascend the *second* Time.

To check the *first* Descent.   Pounds. Ounces.
Ballast, at twice: - - - -   24   0
To clear Trees and Hedges, and
  re-ascend:
Barometer and Frame, - - -   0   12½

sons in Motion towards him, who proved to be several *Farmers* and *Labourers* who had run themselves out of Breath to *overtake* the Balloon.

One asked the Aironaut, whether he intended to alight; and was answered, " *Not for any Time.*"

Proof of the gentle Descent.

100. The Car alighted each Time so *smoothly*, that neither the *Watch* nor *Thermometer* that lay near each other on the *green* Bays at the Bottom, were displaced. Nor was the *Glass Tube* containing the Quicksilver, separated from the Division of the Frame in which it was originally fixed: but the whole was brought back, a few Days after, in a perfect State: except

	lb.	oz.
Basket with Tunning Dish and Bottles (except the Flask with Brandy and Water) - - -	4	10
Half Mile of Twine on the Reel	1	0
Speaking Trumpet - - - -	0	$8\frac{1}{2}$
Woollen Gloves - - - - -	0	1
	31	0
	24	0
Remains for Re-ascent	7	0

except a small Hole, made in Consequence of the inverted Situation of the *Mercury* in Vacuo, *which* fell against the Top of the exhausted Tube.

 The Car *first* landed at 28 Minutes past III, in a Field belonging to a Farm called Bellair, in the Township of Kingsley, near two Miles East by South from the Town of Frodsham, and twelve from Chester.

<small>Balloon landed near Frodsham.</small>

END OF THE FIRST PART.

(c) To find the Length of the Shadow at half paſt III.
(See Section 84, Note *a*.)

Given { Lat. of Cheſter, - 53° 12′
Sun's Dec. - - 5 29 } To find Sun's Alt.
Hour III. 30M. - 52 30 }

This is the Caſe of an oblique ſpheric Triangle, wherein are two Sides and one Angle between them given, to find the Sun's Azimuth, and the Sun's Co-Alt.

Side - - - 84. 31 } Sum of Sides - - 121. 19
Side - - - 36. 48 } Diff. of Sides - 47. 43
(3½ Hour) Angle contained - 52. 30
Half ditto - - - - 26. 15 } 63. 45
Half Sum of Sides - - - 60. 39 } Co. 29. 22
Half Difference ditto - - 23. 51 } 66. 9

THE FIRST PREPARATIVE PROPORTION.

As Sine of ½ Sum of Sides - - - - 60. 39   0.05966 Co-
To Sine of ½ Difference of Sides - - 23. 51   9.60675 Ar.
So Co-Tangent ½ contained Angle - 63. 45   10.30703

To T. of ½ Diff. of the other two Angles 43. 15   9.97344

SECOND PREPARATIVE PROPORTION.

As Co-Sine ½ Sum of Sides - - - 29. 21   0.30968 Co-
To Co-Sine ½ Diff. - - - - - 66. 9   9.96123 Ar.
So Co-Tangent ½ contained Angle - 63. 45   10.30703

To T. ½ Sum of other Angles - - 75. 11 10.57794
Half Diff. before found - - - 43. 15

Sum, is greater Angle - - - 118. 26 = Sun's Azim.
Diff. is leſſer Angle - - - - 31. 56 = S's right Aſc.

Then by firſt Axiom in Trigonometry, to know the Sun's Altitude ſay,

As Sine Sun's right Aſc. - - - - 31. 56   0.27659
To Sine Co-Lat. - - - - - - 36. 48   9.77744
So Sine of the contained Angle - - 52. 30   9.89947

To Co-Sine of the Sun's Alt. - - 63. 57   9.95350
     from 90.

Sun's Alt. - - - - 26. 3

Having Sun's Alt. to find the Shadow,

As Sine Sun's Alt. - - - - 26. 3   0.35738 Co-Ar.
To Perſon's Height, - - - 66 *Inches*, 1.81954
So Co-Sine of the Sun's Alt. - 63. 57   9.95350

To Length of Shadow, - - 135 *Inches*, 2.13042

Then $6(\frac{66}{135} = \frac{11}{22}) - \frac{3}{6}$ or $\frac{1}{2}$, i. e. as 22 to 45: ſuppoſing the Length of the Shadow divided into 45 Parts; the *Height* of the Object woud be 22 of thoſe Parts; or not quite *half* the *Length* of the Shadow, at half paſt III.

AIROPAIDIA.

THE SECOND PART

OF AN

AËRIAL EXCURSION

FROM CHESTER THE EIGHTH OF SEPT. 1785.

CHAPTER XVIII.

RE-ASCENT OF THE BALLOON.

Section 101. BELLAIR - Meadow: half paſt III o'Clock: *(a)* Thermom. at 55 : *bright* Sun : *few* Clouds in Sight.

The Balloon being now 31 Pound lighter; taking a Direction FROM the Sea-Breeze into the Country, and *again* towards Aſton-Hall *(b)* ; mount- ed

Balloon rapidly re-aſcending.

(a) The Sun's Azimuth from the North Point *Weſtward*, being 118°.26′ : its Supplement to 18c° is 61°.34′ South weſterly : i. e. South Weſt by Weſt, half Weſt *nearly*.

(b) The *Length* of the Shadows being more than *double* the Height of the OBJECTS; ſee *(c)*.

ed up like a Sky-Rocket, with accelerating Velocity: its upper Parts *nodding* from Side to Side, as if to *shake off* the *resisting* Column of Air immediately above it.

<small>The Neck tyed.</small>

102. There being no proper Opportunity of closing the Mouth of the Balloon on its *near* Approach to the Sea, or during the *Swiftness* of its Descent; tho' there had been *frequent Inclination* to attempt it; this *little* but ESSENTIAL Work was instantly resolved upon. And the more so, as the Mouth had continued open *from* the first: and as Mr. Lunardi did not *happen* to mention this Circumstance:

<small>Drawing the Valve, while Mouth of the Balloon is open, shewn to be *dangerous*.</small>

the Utility of which, tho' *too late* to be put in Practice, had, but a few Minutes before, very plainly suggested itself. His Directions were, to *open* the Valve in order to descend: which woud *possibly* have *encreased* the Rapidity of Descent: and, by *introducing* a thorou' Air *upwards*, while the Motion of the Balloon was in a *contrary* Direction,

rection, might have occasioned a *dangerous Rupture* of the lower Parts of the Balloon, *which* actually took Place in a preceding Excursion.

103. The Balloon, tho' rising *quick*, seemed *not* to be wholly disengaged from the Ground, but to have received a Check; and to *lean* a little out of the Perpendicular: particularly the Car, which was evidently drawn a *different* Way *from* the Balloon. *The Balloon drawn sideways.*

On perceiving that the half Mile *white* Flag, fastened to the *upper* Hoop of the Car, sensibly impeded the Elevation of the Machine, by *trailing* along the Ground, (the Balloon being yet within the Influence of the Sea-Breeze, or *lower* Current of Air;) the Question was, whether it woud not be imprudent to suffer the Balloon to rise near half a Mile, before the *white* Flag was *disentangled* and free to follow it. *The half Mile white Flag impeding the Balloon.*

For as neither the *Twine*, nor the *lower Cords* of the Balloon were of Silk; the Twine having lain on the Trees

Trees or MOIST Ground, might become a CONDUCTOR from the Earth to any Stratum of Air that had LESS or MORE than what is called its natural Quantity *(a)* of the ELECTRIC Fluid.

Twine cut, left it fhoud prove a Conductor of Electricity.

Adding to the above, a Wifh to rife higher the *second* Time than the firft; ftooping for the Sciffars, the String was *cut:* referving a Remainder to tye the Neck of the Balloon; which was immediately done by gathering the Parts of the Balloon into the Hand, wrapping a Couple of Yards loofely round, and tying them on a SLIP or BOW Knot: one End of which was PURPOSELY left hanging three Feet downwards, to *untye* inftantly on Occafion.

Additional Levity of one Pound.

This additional Levity of *nearly* one Pound, gave the whole Quantity of Ballaft thrown over in a *few* Minutes, *nearly* 32 Pounds.

Remarks on the Balloon.

104. The intelligent Farmer who ftood near the Balloon, when it alighted at Bellair, had obferved it for fome Time *before* near the Sea, and marked its

---

(a) See " Prieftley on Electricity."

its Return, as coming *apparently* from *Overton*.

At firſt, which was *more* than five Minutes before it came to the Ground, it ſeemed to him as if it coud not have been *larger* than a Bladder.

He ſaw it reaſcend, firſt *ſideways*, then upright; moving from the Sea.

Afterward it roſe *rapidly*, and rather *towards* the Sea and Warrington, diſtant twelve Miles.

He watched it for a Quarter of an Hour: and caught it by Intervals, near and above a Cloud in the *blue* Sky, at ſo great a Height that it looked like a *Lark*: and at laſt ſo *ſmall* that the People who ſtood near him coud none of them regain a *Sight*, when they had once loſt it.

Apparent Size of the Balloon, when ſeen from *below*.

105. The remaining *white* Flag was unfolded, and tyed to one of the Balloon-Cords attached to the *upper* Hoop, at a proper Diſtance to *play* freely in the Wind: and, notwithſtanding all that has been ſaid to the contrary

contrary, shewed *instantaneously* and *plainly* the corresponding Changes made by the Wind in different Directions.

And, as the Breeze was accompanied with a Sensation of *Coolness* against the Face of the Aironaut, looking towards that Quarter from whence the Wind came, as indicated by the Flag; (which Quarter was not in a Line with the Path of the Balloon;) the Flag must have shewn that the Change was made by the *Air* in *its peculiar* progressive Direction, and not by *its* Resistance or Progress in the Track of the Balloon.

Balloon moving in a Direction different from that of the Air.

106. It is probable that the *Momentum* of the Balloon, acquired by its centrifugal or accelerating Force upwards, might have kept it in *one* Direction, while it continued to rise throu' *different* Currents.

CHAP-

CHAPTER XIX.

BALLOON STILL RE-ASCENDING.

Section 107. THE Balloon being now *wholly* uncon- fined, continued to *rise* with *great* Rapidity: croffed the Meadow in the Sea-Breeze, and remained as *before*, for 6 or 8 Minutes,—by Intervals *gently* turning on its Axis—almoft wholly *vertical* over Afton-Hall, but rather more to the *Eaftward* of it. Balloon vertical over Afton, for 8 Minutes.

The Country ftill exhibited *bright gay* and EXTENSIVE Profpects.

108. *Three* Sail of *Veffels* appeared in the CHANNEL: and *four more* were failing down the River Wever, *apparently* juft under the Balloon, diminifhing to *mere Cockle-Shells*, or like *Boats* which have *no* Rigging.

Shouts continued.

Corn and Cattle were vifible in the Fields and Meadows.

Afton, tho' a *large* and *elegant Manſion*, appeared like a *Houſe* which Children *build* with *Cards*.

<small>Chillineſs felt at the ſame Height in re-aſcending.</small>

109. A Chillineſs in the Air was again perceived in riſing, as he imagined, to the *ſame* Height at which he felt it in *deſcending*, indicated by the Thermometer at 55°. (Sect. 92.)

He then found himſelf inclined to taſte the *Brandy and Water*, ready mixed by his Order, and to eat a Biſcuit: but on putting the Liquor to his Lips; thought it *too* ſtrong, ſo drank none, nor eat any Thing.

110. The *three* Sail, and the *Channel diſappeared*.

<small>River *red*.</small>

The River put on a deep *red* Colour, like the Dee. Its Meanders ſeemed to *encreaſe*; as its Width *diminiſhed* to a *broad* Line. Its Water was *loſt* to the Sight.

Corn and Cattle were no longer diſtinguiſhable.

The Houſe at Afton was yet a beautiful tho' minute Object: the Balloon

loon moving several Times round it; as if loth to quit *that* and the River.

The Cascade was become a *white* Line: and the *fine* Bridge below, a *yellow Straw* crossing the broad *red* Streak.

Of the *four* Vessels in the Wever, *not* an *Atom* visible.

The Shouting entirely ceased.

111. The *blue* scattered Houses, wide public Road called Sutton-Causeway over Frodsham Marsh, the Meadows Fields and Woods, the *lofty* Hills, Helsbye Crag and Halton-Tower, were *reduced* to *one common* Level; and diminished to the Size and Semblance of a *coloured* Map, but it was the *superb* and *finished* Colouring of NATURE. Rocks Woods and Meads reduced to a *coloured Plain* of the *mellowest* Tints.

112. Ceasing to look *down* on the smooth LAWNS *below*, which were *now* of the richest and *fullest* Patterns, seen as thro' the *small* or inverted End of a common Perspective-Glass, and *spun*, as it were, to a *fine Thread*; Pleasure Balloon higher than at the *first* Ascent.

P 2   and

and Delight, tho' of another Kind, fill'd the Imagination of the Beholder: who, raising his Eyes on a Level with himself, so as to look *straight before* him; found that the Balloon had *already*, and almost beyond his own Belief, soared to so amazing a Height in the Atmosphere, as to raise him *far* above the RIM of the immense Bowl or Crater; and that it was still *stealing* with *Rapidity* upwards.

Contemplation of the Prospect. 113. During the Contemplation of this magnificent Prospect, a *perfect* Calm took Place, and *soothing Silence* reigned.

And thus; for *a while* detached, *far* detached from Earth, and *all* terrestrial Thoughts; wrapt in the *mild Azure* of the *etherial* Regions; suspended in the Center of a vast and almost endless Concave; come, as a *mere* VISITOR, from *another* Planet; surrounded with the stupendous Works of *Nature*, yet *above* them;—the GLORIOUS SUN except, which enlivened ALL, and shone with

with pure celestial Lustre;—a peaceful SERENITY of *Mind* succeeded; an ENVIABLE EUROIA. *(a)* An Idea of which it is not in the Power of Language to convey, or to describe.

CHAPTER XX.

Section 114. Respiration at so great an Altitude was perfectly free and *easy*: *forced* Trials being made for Information on that Point: a Sensation of Levity seemed *rather* to be communicated by the Air to the Lungs: but this might be the Effect of the Imagination. It was however a *curious* Circumstance to find the Breath *not* visible; the Thermometer rising AGAIN to 60. Nor did the Pulse seem to be quicker than *usual*, in this elevated tho' *inactive* Situation.

Breathed freely. Thermometer 60.

115. The

(a) Ἐυροια.

Thunder-Clouds as before.

115. The Perspective of a vast Series of Thunder-Clouds of a *sulphureous* and *metallic* Tinge, placing themselves in Ranks, each beyond the other, in *bright* and tremendous Order, and a Sort of *Battle-Array*, beyond Conception grand yet *beautiful*; coud not pass *under* him without Notice. The immense circular and visible Distance of the NEBULOUS Horizon, extended NOW 102 Miles *at the least* round the Eye, as already mentioned (Sect. 52); was a grand Source of the Sublime.

Fairy Landscapes striking.

Nor did the contracted View of the Landscape below fail, in Turn, to *regain* an Attention to its *indiscriminate* yet *pleasing* Scenery.

116. ON A SUDDEN he was called back to himself.

Bladders crackling.

Several of the BLADDERS, which were tyed round the Car, in Case the Balloon shoud *alight on* the Sea, and were DRY on the Outside, began at the same Instant to CRACKLE; being greatly distended by the Air within.

When

When preſſed with the Hands and Fingers, they felt extremely hard, and *ready* to *burſt*.

On looking upwards at the Balloon, it appeared GREATLY inflated: the external Preſſure of the ſurrounding Air being *much leſſened*, in ſo elevated and *rarified* a State of the Atmoſphere. *Balloon bloated.*

117. The Balloon *preſſed* in an unuſual Manner *throu'* the Meſhes of the Net, quite round. *Balloon quilted by internal Preſſure.*

118. The Shape was much altered by this Diſtention of the Sides: and its *perpendicular* Diameter *ſhorter* than before. *Balloon ſhorter and broader.*

119. The Neck or *Mouth*, which was *tyed*, had actually riſen *upwards*, and was THEN near *eight* Feet above the Bottom of the *Car*. *Neck 8 Feet above the Car.*

120. It was not known till afterwards, that Mr. Lunardi on his ſecond aërial Voyage from Liverpool, had been obliged to cut off the *lower* Part of the *Neck*, weighing upwards of *two* Pounds and a *half*, in order to lighten his *Neck cut off in a former Excurſion.*

his Defcent near *Tarporley* in Che-fhire; and that he had not *Silk* fuffi-cient to repair the Lofs.

CHAPTER XXI.

An Attempt to reach the Twine by climbing on the Car.

Section 121. IN vain did the Aironaut ftrive to reach the *Neck* of the Balloon, from the *Car*. Attempting to put his Feet on the *oppofite* Sides of the *lower* Hoop, by grafping the *upper* with his Hands; he coud not in *that* Situation raife himfelf fo high *as before*; nor let go his Hold with *either* Hand.

He then ftepped *down* into the *Car*. The Agitation of *which*, brought within the Reach of his Hand, the loofe *End* of the Twine *(purpofely tyed on a Bow or Slip Knot)* that had ftuck to one of the Side-Cords, and held the *Center* of the *Neck* rather *out* of the Perpendicular.

CHAP-

CHAPTER XXII.

BALLOON AT ITS GREATEST HEIGHT.

Section 122. **B**Eing cautious how he suffered the LIGHT-EST Gafs to efcape throu' the Top of the Balloon, which muft have happened in drawing down the String of the Valve; yet apprehending the POSSIBILITY of an immediate Rupture at its PRESENT GREATEST Elevation;—glancing his Eyes *around* to take a FAREWEL View;—he *pulled* the Twine, that tyed the NECK. *[Mouth of the Balloon opened.]*

123. *Inftant* Relief was given to the Balloon: which fhrunk into the Shape which it had affumed in the former Afcent, when the Gafs began to iffue in vifible Vapour, the *Neck* likewife *lowering* itfelf to the Height of his Shoulders, as in Section 35. *[Balloon for to its ufual Shape.]*

124. On ftooping he found the Time 41 Minutes after III, and the Thermometer 57. *[Mouth opened at 41 Minutes paft III.]*

Q   Nor

No visible Vapour escaped.

Nor was he surprised that no *visible* Vapour escaped; as he had imagined that much *common* Air had been pressed into the *Mouth* of the Balloon: and which, being *heavier* than Gass, woud *go out first.*

Why the Valve at the Top is not to be opened.

On that Ground he was confirmed in his Resolution *not* to open the Valve at the Top, which always emits the *lightest* Gass.

The Neck being made Air-tight, the Balloon rose again.

125. As soon however as the Neck of the Balloon reached his Shoulder, he *gathered* the Silk in his Hand, and held it *Air-tight* tho' untyed, to prevent Evaporation of much *real* Gass: presuming that if any Levity remained; the Balloon woud presently *rise* again, and *swell.*

And he was pleased to find the Event answer his Expectations.

CHAP.

CHAPTER XXIII.

AIR WARMER ABOVE THAN BELOW.

Section 126. IT was a Matter both of Surprize and Pleasure to observe that the Thermometer had risen AGAIN to 60, when the Balloon had soared *above* the Sea-Breeze; as the Aironaut had expected to feel the extreme Rigour of Winter; and had made Preparations against *intense* Cold.

Nor did he find any Difficulty in Respiration *during* the Excursion; which may possibly be accounted for from the *Warmth* of the Air.

That the Breath *(a)* was *not* visible at any one Time, and particularly while the

The Breath not visible during the Excursion.

(a) The Breath is said to become *visible* at Sea or Land at any Temperature of the Thermometer not *exceeding* 60°: tho', in Latitude 41°, and Westward of the Azores Islands, being in Sight of the Peak of ST. GEORGE, (which probably equals, if not exceeds, the Height of Teneriffe) the Observer has seen his *own Breath*, and *that* of the Sailors on Deck, when the Thermometer in the *Shade* was at 61: the Air (in January) being *then remarkably* damp.

An Account of the Breath being visible at Sea, when the Thermometer was at 61.

the Balloon was elevated above the *under* Current, might it not be owing to the uncommon DRYNESS of the Air, which woud *diſſipate* the Vapour at the Inſtant of *Expoſure?*

<small>Encreaſed Shadows ſeem to raiſe the Objects.</small>

127. It was remarked, ſome little Time *before*, and *during* the *laſt* Glance of the Proſpect taken at the *higheſt* Elevation, that the Houſe at Aſton was ſtill viſible, and the *dark coloured* LINE forming its DIMINUTIVE Shadow ſeemed *thicker* in Proportion to the *Plan*, than when the Manſion was *firſt* ſeen before the Re-aſcent. And it had a *ſenſible* Effect in *apparently raiſing* it above the *common* Level.

<small>Proſpects below noted.</small>

128. The Circuit of the *Land-Abyſs below* was alſo greatly *contracted*: and a Hazineſs inclining to a *dark Green* ſeemed to cover the *outward* Verge round the *Lawn*.

The *red* River Wever only appeared.

The Channel and *broad* Branch of the

the River Merſey towards Warrington, had long ſince vaniſhed.

The Lawn itſelf, which compoſed the Ground-View, was full of *innumerable* Encloſures *almoſt* CLOSE to each other; with *much* Wood :— dwindling to the Pattern of an elegant Turkey-Carpet : which, according to Principles of Mahommedan Faith, tho' wrought in *gay* and *vivid* Colours, is *made* to exhibit NO EXACT *(a)* Reſemblance to the Works either of Art or Nature.

<small>*Down* View like the Pattern of a Turkey-Carpet.</small>

129. The Colours, of which the Ground Work was *principally* formed (except WHITE; alſo the *roughened* Sea, which *alone* was BLACK; and Shadows, which *conſtantly* gave a *tranſparent* VIOLET) were four ſimple and *primary* ones, viz. RED, YELLOW, GREEN, and BLUE: all which ſeemed

<small>The Earth *glowing* with *primary* Colours only.</small>

(a) This Aſſertion may ſeem to contradict what was ſaid in Section 44: When—" every Thing, that coud be ſeen at all, was ſeen DISTINCT:" but it only proves that the Balloon had attained a greater Altitude during the Re-aſcent, and that the SHADOWS were *much lengthened*, as the Evening advanced.

ed to GLOW, tho' in a *less* Degree, like the Colours of the Prism.

This unmixed *Coloration* of Objects, from a vertical Situation *only*, to be seen without *Refraction*, is a new singular and *pleasing* Phenomenon.

Cromatic View of the Earth, an Appearance peculiar to the Balloon.

130. A View, taken *above* the Level of the Clouds, may, from this Circumstance, without Impropriety, be called a CHROMATIC VIEW of the Earth: of which, the *Print* is an Example: delineating the Extent of the aërial Excursion; and placed at the End of the *second* Part, including the Re-ascent.

CHAPTER XXIV.

BALLOON ABOVE THE INFLUENCE OF WATER.

Balloon above the Influence of the Waters and Sea-Breeze.

Section 131. THE Balloon pursued its former *gentle* Course in the *upper* Current of Air moving from the South West, and Aston

Afton House: and had rifen *above* the Influence of the *Waters* and *Sea-Breeze.*

132. In Confequence of having *held tight* the Neck of the Balloon, the Gafs *within* began *again* to expand, and the Machine became *more bloated* than when *ftationary* at the firft Afcent: the Bottom of the Balloon being drawn up to the Height of his Hand, when the Arm was ftretched, and himfelf on Tip-toe. Balloon repeatedly fwelling.

133. Tho' the late Defcent, at the laft OPENING of the Balloon, had been rapid; which was known *chiefly* by the Want of Reaction from the Bottom of the Car againft the Soles of the Feet; yet being ftill *far above all* Clouds; fearlefs of the *Currents, Rocks,* and *Shoals,* to which ALL MARITIME *Navigation* is fubject; he took the Opportunity of trying the upper Valve; *purpofely* to know the Effect. So retaining the Bottom of the Balloon The Valve firft tried.

in his *right* Hand, he drew the Valve Cord with his *left*.

Immediately he heard it *click*: which proved that it was quite open, and in good Order.

<small>The Valve anſwered.</small>

134. He tried the Valve three Times *ſmartly*, and deliberately.

The Eſcape of the inflammable Air or Gaſs was like the *growling* Sound made in a Mill by the Grinding of the Mill-ſtones, but by no Means ſo loud.

CHAPTER XXV.

THIRD BALLOON-IRIS.

<small>Balloon-Shadow.</small>

Section 135. THE *ſucceſſive* Operations of untying the Neck, and *repeated* Trials of the Valve, brought the Obſerver ſo low, that he coud trace the *Image* of the Balloon on the *upper* Surface of *light ſilvery* Clouds beneath him.

136. *Iris*

136. *Iris*, a bright *celestial* Nymph, his *former* Attendant, deck'd in gay Attire as usual for the Bow, made her *third* Appearance: instantly *encircling* the Balloon. Nor was her Stay so short as before; as if to *recompense* the Aironaut for the lost Sight of Earth and all *terrestrial* Objects, which then began to *disappear*. Third Balloon. Iris.
Iris remained.
The Earth disappeared.

137. In less than *a Minute* after the *Deflation*; the Neck of the Balloon continuing to be held tight in the Hand; the Balloon *quickly* encreased in Bulk, and soared *aloft*, as before.

138. It continued *rising* as long as the Hand coud *reach* to hold the Neck tight: and, on loosing it *an Instant*, made a rapid Descent: on Account of the *Gass* which escaped, and of the atmospheric *Air* which rushed in by the *same* Opening at the Bottom. Balloon alternately rising and falling.

139. The alternate Play of FAST AND LOOSE, was frequently and *successfully* repeated: the Balloon always rising till it swelled out of the Reach The Play of *fast and loose* repeated.

of the Hand: at which Time it was let go: and the Neck (as well as the Balloon) defcending; was *prefently* caught in the Hand, and made *Air-tight* as before.

<small>Manouvres feen at the Diftance of 15 Miles.</small>

140. Thefe Manouvres were performed, at a Height *far* above the Level of *all* Clouds, and in Sight of Numbers of People: fome of whom were at leaft 15 Miles diftance: yet coud plainly, from an Eminence called *Hoole-Mill* Field, a Couple of Miles from Chefter, difcover the Balloon at an amazing Height, darting up and down feveral Times; or as they expreffed themfelves, " *quivering and warping in the Air.*"

CHAPTER XXVI.

SENSATIONS ACCOMPANYING THE BALLOON.

<small>Situation fafe and pleafant.</small>

Section 141. THE alternate Elevation and Defcent of the Balloon gave fufficient Leifure to reflect on the SECURITY and PLEASURE of

of his Situation, thus *wafted* on the *Pinions*, and *merging* in the *Ocean* of Air.

Indeed the whole Excursion was a continued Scene of Pleasure.

The Eye and the Imagination were beyond Measure delighted.

142. If there had been any Thing to wish for, it was the *living* Pencil of ANGELICA, (*b*) or some other celebrated Painter: in order to gratify the World with the *bright Miniatures* and *Colouring* of so much *variegated* Beauty.

143. As it woud be difficult, if not impossible, by *mere* Description, to convey an adequate Idea of the different SENSATIONS experienced while in the Car; (for Pleasure is itself unspeakable;) yet the Fancy may possibly, without Censure, be a Moment *indulged*, in its Allusions to such familiar Subjects as approach nearest to THEM: so as not to leave the *public* Mind *wholly* in the Dark, with Respect to the above Points of natural and general Curiosity.

(*b*) Angelica Kauffman.

The Swing a favourite Amusement.

144. Moſt young People, whenever they have Opportunity, amuſe themſelves on the SLACK ROPE, or Swing: the Pleaſure *encreaſes* in Proportion to the *Loftineſs of Aſcent* they are *able* to acquire.

The Mogul enjoys the Air without Fatigue, by Means of the Swing.

145. In the Eaſt, where the Heat of the Climate forbids robuſt Exerciſes; the *Swing* is conſidered as a princely Diverſion: and of which the MOGUL himſelf *condeſcends* to partake. He is ſwung by Slaves: and thus enjoys the *pure* Air *without* Fatigue.

The Balloon and Swing compared.

146. The Aſcent of the Balloon is not unlike what is felt, in the *aſcending* half of the Swing: and the Deſcent is attended with that agreeable Senſation known to thoſe who *ſink* throu' the *deſcending* half.

A favourite Diverſion among the Ruſſians.

147. A Diverſion ſimilar to the above is peculiar to the *North of Europe*, practiſed by the Ruſſians, particularly the Inhabitants of Zarſko Zelo; and accompanied with a Senſation *ſo delightful*,

lightful, that they seek it in the *open* Air, amidst the *utmost Severity* of the *Frost*. It is a Sort of Boat or *Car*, in which they *glide*, for a considerable Distance, *down* an *artificial* Declivity of *waved* and *polished* Ice: being drawn up by Servants; they launch precipitately forwards, and *down* again as before. Artificial Declivity of *waved* Ice.

148. *Sledges* drawn *swiftly* over the undulated Surface of a *snowy* Country, is a favourite Diversion in many Parts of Germany, in Lapland, and Siberia: Skaiting on *level* Ice; the Motion of a Vessel on *smooth* Water; of a *fleet* Horse; also of Wheel-Carriages rolling over EVEN Gravel, or a *grassy* Plain, are each a *Luxury* of the same Kind; and *grateful* to the Nerves. Amusements of Gestation in common with the Balloon.

149. There is yet another Amusement, which is said to be of *German* Extraction, still frequent in the North of England, called the *vertical* FLYING-COACH. (*a*) Vertical Flying-Coach.

Two

(*a*) It consists of a Frame, made by placing

Two Perſons are required to turn the Machine (when full): which moves like the four Sails of a Wind-mill: a Seat being placed at the End of each Sail.

150. The *Pleaſure* communicated to the Nerves *during* the Deſcent, is to ſome Conſtitutions ſo *exquiſite*, as to be full as much as the human Frame can ſupport: others are affected by it in a *gentler* Manner.

Theſe different Diverſions, flowing from the ſame Principle in common with the Balloon, viz. that of *being carried with a gentle Motion*, are *one or other* ſuited to all Ranks and Ages.

151. The two ſtrong Poſts, moveable at Pleaſure, each nine or ten Feet high, upright in the Ground, at the Diſtance of two Yards: the Poſts being well ſecured by broad Pedeſtals, to keep them firm: a ſtrong horizontal Iron Axis goes throu' the Top of the Poſts; and throu' the Centers of four Arms or Levers at their Junction.

Between the four correſponding Ends of each two Arms, (which Arms are alſo ſtrengthened by Beams from one to the other), are fixed four Seats or Boxes, well ſecured, each holding three or four Perſons, and moving on Iron Pivots, near the Top of the Boxes, ſo as always to preſerve the *vertical* Equilibrium.

151. The Pleasure of the double Slack Ropes, when seated in the Car appended between them, is perhaps in itself *superior* to that of most others.

152. The *vertical Flying-Coach* (*a*) compleats the *Circle*, of which the Slack Rope describes but the lower *Half*.

153. The Sensations communicated by the Motion of the Balloon, come nearest those of the vertical flying Coach, tho' *more* gentle, and if possible, *more* pleasing. {*Balloon and Vertical Flying-Coach compared.*}

At Sea, the most experienced Mariner is sometimes *sick* or *giddy*. {*No Sickness or Giddiness in the Balloon.*}

154. Nothing of the Kind happens in the Balloon: where an infinite Variety charms the Imagination.

155. The Spirits are raised by the *Purity* of the Air (*c*), and *rest* in a *chearful* Composure. {*The Spirits raised.*}

Even

(*a*) Why not recommend the Use of that Machine to Invalids? who woud find Refreshment in the OPEN Air: as its Rotation communicates a gentle Motion to the System, (*b*) without the least Fatigue; *rather* encreasing the *Animal* Spirits. {*Recommended to Invalids.*}

(*b*) Particularly the Stomach and Diaphragm. See " Berdoe's Enquiry."

(*c*) Talis Aër qualis Spiritus. See " *Health's Improvement*," by Dr. Moffet, Chapter 3, Of Air, Page 79.

The greateſt Height conveys no Fear of falling.

156. Even when *ſtationary* above the Clouds, the *Height* conveys with it no *Danger* of *falling:* any more than *when* in a Veſſel at Sea, (as off the Weſt-India Iſlands, for Example) the *Fiſh* are ſeen gliding over the clear *white rocky* Bottom, at the Depth of twenty Fathom: as the Aironaut ſeems perfectly unconnected with the Earth, and unconcerned about it.

The Depth below the Clouds gives no Idea of Diſtance.

157. Nor does the Depth *below the Clouds* give an Idea of *Diſtance*. On the contrary, the *ſmooth chequered Lawns* which form the Surface of the Earth, are preſented to the Eye, as on a *Level* with the *Clouds* themſelves: *at leaſt* COME UP to their UNDERSIDES, and appear ſo much a Part of *them*; that the *Clouds* occupy the Place of *Earth:* and the Aironaut ſeems able to deſcend from the *Car* upon the *Clouds,* and to walk from Side to Side over the *empty* Space, as over a Sheet of *tranſparent* Ice, acroſs a *River*, whoſe Depth is equal to the *ſmall* but indefinite Thickneſs of the Clouds.

158. It

158. It is from *frequent* EXPERIENCE only that the *Diminution of Objects* presuppose their *Distance*.

CHAPTER XXVII.

USEFUL CONCLUSIONS.

Section 159. IT was remarkable that the lower Parts of the Balloon regularly adopted a *similar* Form at each Descent: not unlike a *Ship's Bottom*; looking up at the Head or Prow, while on the Stocks: the *Neck* of the Balloon forming a beautiful *central* Pillar; in Shape like that of a *Speaking Trumpet* inverted.

<small>Change in the *Form* of the Balloon while descending: with Conclusions drawn from the Change.</small>

And hence may be derived a Piece of *useful* Information: as the *precise* Time of descending is discovered by bare *Inspection* of the Machine.

<small>Time of Descent discovered by the Form of the Balloon.</small>

160. Another Conclusion seems likewise deducible from the above, that if the

<small>Balloon adopting the Form of an elliptic Solid.</small>

the Balloon is so burdened, as to *descend* while it retains the Form of an ELLIPTIC SOLID; *(a)* it will descend more rapidly, than if it contained less Gass: the Force of Descent in both Cases being supposed the same.

For if the Diminution of Gass be so great as *not* to fill the upper Hemisphere of the *Balloon*; the Resistance of the atmospheric Air *below* woud probably give *it* the Appearance of a *Concave* or Umbrella, which woud greatly *check* the Descent: viz. in Proportion to the Square of the Number of Feet of which the Surface was composed.

161. Hence also the evident Utility of an EQUATORIAL HOOP for Balloons: in Preference to a Parashute, which woud be only an Incumbrance.

An equatorial Hoop preferred to a Parashute.

CHAP.

(a) Or Solid of *least* RESISTANCE, see Chambers's Dictionary, with the Supplement.

CHAPTER XXVIII.

Section 162. AT 40 Minutes paſt III, when the Balloon was *apparently* ſome Miles above the Level and Summit of the Clouds; a SUDDEN and uncommon *Sound* was heard for three or four Seconds only. *An uncommon Sound in the Air.*

A Sort of *hollow* Wind ſeemed iſſuing from a Plain of Clouds in the North-Eaſt Quarter, greatly below the Balloon: which as SUDDENLY ceaſed.

The Inſtant the Sound was heard; a gentle Motion was *impreſſed* on the Balloon, as if by a Hand touching *it* near the *Top*. *An unuſual Motion communicated to the Balloon.*

163. Clouds to the North-Eaſt appeared, for the firſt Time, in *rapid* Motion towards the Balloon.

They *ſailed* directly *under* it: filled up the Chaſm, and drew a *white* Veil over *all terreſtrial* Objects.

164. It has been *ſince* imagined, that

Conjecture in the Caufe of the Motion. a frefh Wind *defcended* from the South-Weft Quarter in the upper Current, and was heard in the North-Eaft, being ecchoed from the upper Tier of Clouds *below*: and that the Balloon, finding lefs Refiftance than the RANGE of Clouds, foon overtook and paffed them: particularly as the lower Part of the *white* Flag vibrated only in the ufual Direction.

165. The *encreafed* progreffive Motion of the Balloon was *not* perceived (Section 18): being confidered as at *Reft*, and the *apparent* Motion *referred* to the *Clouds*.

CHAPTER XXIX.

Section 166. IN a few Minutes, a Side-Break throu' the Clouds difcovered a long ill-formed narrow Line or Ditch, fomething lefs than a Foot in Breadth, extending feveral several Ways: and which from its Proximity to Places that were known, and coming into View; viz. the Country about Norton and Halton-Castle; proved to be the Duke of Bridgewater's Canal.

<small>A narrow Ditch the Duke of Bridgewater's Canal.</small>

SUDDENLY came in Sight the *spacious* OPEN of the Mersey above Runcorn Gap: which appeared of a RUDDY Colour, and *very* near: as if the Balloon had again *felt* the Influence of the *River*.

<small>A Glympse of Runcorn Gap.</small>

167. A new System, that of *Balloon-Geography* here suggested itself: in which the Essentials of *Proportion* and *Bearings* woud be far more accurate, than by the present Method, both for *Maps* and *Charts*, viz. To make Drawings by SIGHT, from the Car of a Balloon with a *Camera Obscura*, aided by a Micrometer applied to the under Side of *the transparent* Glass.

<small>Balloon-Geography first suggested for Maps.</small>

The Season proper for such an aironautic Expedition, would be *any calm*

calm bright Day: the Wind having blown from the South West Quarter, for some Days before, which is *frequently* the Case: the Air, at *such* Conjuncture probably remaining WARM, to the Height of a Mile or more, unless in the very Midst of Winter.

<small>Air presumed to be warm with a South-West Wind long continued.</small>

168. And particularly for Charts, which in a *maritime* Country are *most* useful: as Balloons have an extraordinary Predilection to become *stationary* over Channels and Rivers; altho' a very *strong* Gale of Wind, shoud continue the *whole* Time to blow in an horizontal Course directly UNDER the Balloon.

<small>Balloon Geography for *Charts*.</small>

Of which Event the Writer of this Account was an *Eye-Witness*, in the Case of Mr. Lunardi: who was *detained* above 20 Minutes over the *broad Bend* of the River Mersey, near Ince, in Cheshire, the Day he *landed* between Tarporley and Beeston-Castle, ascending from the New Fort at Liverpool.

<small>Balloon in a Calm with a *strong* Wind *below*.</small>

pool. He quitted his Station by the *Escape* of *Gafs*, and defcended into the *Stream* of Wind, which continued as *violent* as before.

CHAPTER XXX.

Section 169. THE Summer Scenes of Fairy-Land below, being foon eclipfed by the *quick* Intervention of a *Range* of Clouds; the SUDDEN Contraft of which was highly pleafing to the Imagination; a Profpect of MID WINTER inftantaneoufly fucceeded.

170. The Earth's *Surface* feen throu' an immeafurable Crater of Vapour accumulated round the Aironaut, who was fufpended, and feemed fixed in the Center above it, *no longer exifted*. And, if it will not be allowed, that a *new* Earth, and a *new* SKY appeared; at

The Center filled up in an Inftant.

at least, let the Imagery and Resemblance of what was really seen, be taken from that EARTH, which in Fact did *not* appear.

A WORLD of *Clouds*, GREATER than the ONE below, became, for the first Time the *sole* Object that engrossed the Sight. (See Section 144.)

View of the Clouds taken from above *them.*

171. The Balloon was *apparently* raised some Miles above the *Surface* of a *concave shallow* Plate, or Shell, or rather an immense Plain, *which* was in general smooth and well defined: but the *dense* tonitruous Masses, rising here and there *above* the Rest, greatly resembled steep and RUGGED MOUNTAINS seen in Perspective, at different Distances from 5 and 10 to at least a hundred Miles. (*a*)

An unvaried deep cerulean and pellucid

(*a*) It will be found, that, on comparing the *two* Calculations in Section 52, Note (*a*), *corrected*; the circular *Distance* from the Eye, above the Clouds, was 102 Miles, 1 Quarter, 320 Yards: while *that* above the Earth, seen from the same elevated Situation, (supposing the Day to have been CLEAR for such a View,) was 102

lucid Azure, without a Cloud above, enclosed the NOVEL EARTH: whose Surface, whether Valley, Plain, or MOUNTAIN *in Appearance*; seemed as if covered to a prodigious Depth, by successive Falls of Snow, driven and polished by the Winds and Frost, and dazzling to the Sight: the Sun still shining above all, with WHITE, unremitting and invigorating Rays (*a*).

Miles, 1 Quarter, 307 Yards: whose Difference is only 13 Yards: that is, the *Distance* above the Clouds to the *nebulous* Horizon, was *rather* more extensive, than *that* above the Earth to the *terrestrial* Horizon.

It may not, to some Readers, be deemed either unentertaining, or foreign to the Subject; if the Distance of the *Prospect* from the Balloon at its greatest *barometric* Altitude, viz. 2332 Yards, or a Mile and Half within 33 Yards, be compared with the Distance which may be seen from the *Summit* of the principal Mountains in different Parts of the Globe.

1. Cotopàzy, a Mountain in the Province of Quito, in America, and under the equinoctial Line,

---

(*a*) Rays flowing from the Sun seem to be RED ORANGE or YELLOW, according to the Quantity of Vapours floating in the Atmosphere, which absorbs the most refrangible ones: and the fewer the Vapours the more does the Sun's Light approach to a perfect and intense WHITE, according to the Doctrine of Newton: which seems to receive Confirmation from the Purity of the Solar Light, when seen *above Clouds* and *Vapours*, in the Balloon: where the Sun shines not so much with a *golden* as with a *sparkling* SILVER Light.

CHAPTER XXXI.

Brilliant Colouring of dense Clouds,

Section 172. A Thunder Cloud in most grotesque Form;—of superior Magnitude, Density,

Line, is *said* by Ullòa (Vol. 1. Page 422) to be 3126 Toizes or Fathom, i.e. 6252 Yards, or 3 Miles and a Half and 92 Yards in Height.

2. White Mountain, called by the French Mount Blanc, near Geneva, is considered by Sir G. Shuckburgh (Phil. Transf. Vol. 67, Part 2d, Page 598, for the Year 1777) as the highest Land in Europe, Asia, or Africa (known to Europeans) and calculated by him at 5220 Yards, or 3 Miles within 60 Yards above the Level of the Mediterranean Sea.

Monf. Bourit just returned from his last Tour, see his " Defcription de Glacieres" in 1773, makes the White Mountain but 5102 Yards in Height, (which is 30 Yards lower than Teneriffe) including the 410 Yards for the Level of the Lake of Geneva above the Mediterranean.

3. The Peak of Teneriffe in the Canary Islands, which, *in approaching towards it*, Authors agree, may be seen at the Distance of 120 Miles at Sea, if the Weather is clear; (Modern History, Vol. 14th, Page 451;) and, in *returning from it*, is discoverable at the Distance of 150 Miles, according to Glas's History of the Canaries (Page 234);—has been estimated by Dr. Heberden in Madeira (Guide to the Lakes, Page 187) at 5132 Yards, or 3 Miles within 148 Yards.

Glas remarks farther, that in failing from Teneriffe,

A THUNDER CLOUD UNDER THE BALLOON. 139

fity, and BRIGHTNESS—a *celeſtial Colouring*;

T 2

Teneriffe, the Peak, at the Diſtance of 150 Miles is very little darker than the *azure* Sky, on Account of the great Quantity of Vapour intercepted between the Eye and the Mountain: and *not* becauſe it ceaſed to be an Object too ſmall for the Sight; or was in Fact, below the Horizon, and only raiſed by Refraction of the Vapour.

With Reſpect to the Peak of St. George, ſituated in the Iſland called *Pico*, one of the Azòres; the Writer of this Account aſſerts, from the Mouth of an able and experienced Officer in his MAJESTY's *Navy*, who, during the laſt War, cruized ſome Weeks off thoſe Iſlands; that the latter has frequently obſerved the Peak, at the Diſtance of 120 Miles, and coud then diſtinguiſh a *third Part* of its Height *down* the Mountain. Section 126, Note (*a*), ſee alſo (*a*) below.

4. Etna is 3877 Yards above the Mediterranean: (according to Brydone's Tour throu' Sicily

(*a*) As therefore it may be ſuppoſed that the Peak of St. George, in *receding* from it, woud *vaniſh* at the Diſtance of 150 Miles; its Height may *eaſily* be aſcertained geometrically thus:

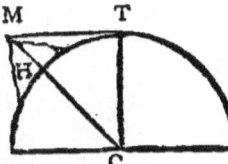

See the Figure annexed.

Let M be the Summit of the Mountain: and let the Line M T drawn to the Circumference of the Circle at T, be the *evaneſcent* Diſtance of the Mountain in the Horizon, viz. 150 Miles.

Join T C, viz. a Line drawn from the *Tangent* to the Center of the Circle, which Line will therefore repreſent the Semidiameter of the *Earth*, viz. 3958 Miles, according to Newton.

Draw a Line from C to M, which will paſs throu' ſome Point of the Circumference as H, the Baſe of the Mountain.

Then, in the Triangle M T C, as the Angle at T is a right Angle (Euclid's Elements, Book 3, Propoſition 18;) and the Sides M T, and T C, containing the right Angle, are *known*; the *third* Side C M is readily found: (being a Corollary to the

47th

louring; and whose *Shade* was itself a Colour of semi-transparent and transcendent

<small>Aironaut lost in the *blue Fields* of Air, by the Intervention of Clouds below him: which prevented all *farther* Knowledge of his Situation, and also a Sight of the Earth itself.</small>

Sicily and Malta, Vol. 1. Page 211) or 2 Miles and 357 Yards.

5. Blue Ridge, the highest Mountain in the Island of Jamaica, is, according to Dr. Clark, who measured it in November last, 3080 Yards, or 1 Mile and three Quarters, above the Level of the Ocean.

The DISTANCE to be SEEN is considered as terminating the Radius of a Circle, whose Center is the EYE of the Observer, on *each* Mountain.

Height of the Mountains.	DISTANCE to be SEEN from them in Miles.
Cotopàzy 3 Miles and a Half and 92 Yards, (for the Process, see Section 52, Note (*a*).	$167\frac{1}{2}$ and 405 Yards.
White Mountain 3 Miles within 60 Yards.	$153\frac{1}{4}$ and 13 Yards.
Peak of Teneriffe 3 Miles within 148 Yards.	152 within 72 Yards.
Mount Etna 2 Miles and 357 Yards.	132 and 127 Yards.
Blue Ridge 1 Mile and 3 Quarters.	$117\frac{3}{4}$ and 30 Yards.
Balloon 1 Mile and half within 33 Yards.	$102\frac{1}{4}$ and 307 Yards.

As it is well known that Objects of the *greatest* Magnitude appear but as BLUE AIR at even a *less* Distance than 100 Miles; to which add the Difficulty

<small>47th Prop. 1st Book Euclid:) viz. having the two Sides of a right Angle Triangle given to find the *third*. Therefore

R U L E.

Multiply the Sides containing the right Angle, each into itself: viz. 150 and 3958: add the Products into one Sum: from which extract the *square Root*; equal to the Length in Miles, of the *third* Side required.

From the *third* Side, subtract that Part, viz. C H, which is</small>

EARTH DISSAPPEARED.

scendent *Blue* and *Violet-Purple* ;—remaining

Difficulty of Journies, and Ascent to the Summit of these astonishing Mounds of Earth; and all this for the Sake, not of a complete DOWN PROSPECT, subject to *a perpetual Variety*, but merely an *imperfect*

is equal to the Semidiameter T C already found: and the Remainder H M is the *Height of the Mountain*.

```
Thus: 150 Miles.      3958 Miles in the Semidiameter of
        150           3958               the Earth.
       ────           ────
       7500           31664
         15           19790
       ────           35622
      22500           11874
Square of the        ───────
greatest visible     15665764 Square of the Semidiameter
Distance.            add 22500     of the Earth.
                     ───────
Extract the sq. Root, 15688264(3960.84 Square Root.
                      9               3958 subtract.
                      ──              ─────
                  69) 668        Rem. 2.84 Answer in Miles.
                      621
                      ───
                  786) 478.2
                       471 6
                       ─────
                79208) 6664.00 continued to 2 Decimals.
                       6336 64
                       ───────
               792164) 32736.00 ditto.
                       31686 56
                       ───────
                         104944
```

To find the .84 Part of a Mile; multiply
1760 Yards in a Mile,
Decimal Parts of a Mile to be reduced .84 into Yards.

```
                              7040
                             14080
                             ─────
                       1760)1478.40(0
             Subtract  1478
                       ────
                         282
```

Answer: the Height of the Mountain is 2 Miles 282 Yards.

maining for several Minutes, *exactly under* the Balloon, *tempted* the Aironaut to descend into it; and, if possible, investigate its Structure and Composition.

Blanchard, he knew, had passed throu' MANY without Danger: any Fears that might otherwise have been entertained on that Head were therefore groundless: particularly as Gass, i. e. *inflammable Air* and the *electric Fluid* (supposing an electric Atmosphere had surrounded the Thunder Cloud) mutually *repel* each other. He however declined the Trial: among other Reasons which then offered; that the temporary and apparent

perfect Side-View: the PLEASURE and EASE of attaining still *more* stupendous Heights at *any* Place and Time, by Means of the BALLOON, are strikingly in Favor of that Invention. And, notwithstanding the confessed Merit of Dr. Black's Project with the *Farciminalis* of a Calf, and Mr. Cavallo's Soap Bubbles with inflammable Air; (see his History of Aerostation, Page 34;) if the Emperor had been alive who offered a Reward for the Invention of a NEW PLEASURE; the *first* Prize had been due to the Brothers Montgolfier, and a *second* to the Brothers Roberts.

rent Reſt of both Balloon and Clouds portended *his* Situation to be over the Center of *ſome Water*: ſo that if *Gaſs* had been let out in order to *deſcend*; *enough* might *not* have remained to make Choice of a proper Place to land.

173. Some Minutes after; on the *Retreat* of the Clouds, or *progreſſive* Motion of the Balloon; he found himſelf ſuſpended over the moſt *enchanting* Meanders of a Rivulet.

Where he coud not tell.

CHAP.

CHAPTER XXXII.

The Aironaut was loft, tho' in Sight of a Country well known when below.

Section 174. HE *thought* himfelf again over the Wever.

At 47 Minutes paft III, over a red Rivulet.

At 47 Minutes after III, the Profpect *beneath* opened, juft wide enough to fhew, that he was fufpended in the open Space over the Center of fome Rivulet.

The Map of the Country which had been fo carefully ftudied, was *now* confulted for the firft Time, but coud not bring to his Recollection any Traces of the extraordinary Curves which then met his Eye.

They bore not the leaft Refemblance to any Part of the River Merfey.

No River like that below him had ever prefented itfelf.

Its *Doublings* were fo various and *fantaftic* as to exceed the Limits of Credibility.

He

175. He was still stationary, at an immense Height, without the *least* Inclination to descend: having *some Time before* taken the Precaution to tye *again* the Neck of the Balloon, as soon as he had perceived it did *not* inflate, as at first, to any *dangerous* Degree.

The Neck of the Balloon tyed some Time before to prevent the Descent.

No Towns, no Houses appeared. No *public Roads* were discoverable. No Voices were heard. (*a*)

U The

(*a*) SOUNDS IMMEDIATELY UNDER the Balloon, seemed, as if originated *near* the Ear, and *louder* than they would have been heard, at the Distance of some Yards *only*, when on a Level with themselves: augmenting rather than decreasing, during the *Ascent* of the Balloon, till it arrived to a Height indicated by the Barometer at 27 Inches. Presently afterwards, the Balloon still rising; the Sounds *died away:* much sooner indeed than was expected.

The like was observed in *descending* from a State of perfect Tranquillity and Silence: *Sounds* from *below*, when about the same Height, *suddenly rushing* on the Ear.

It must be considered that by *this* Time, the SHADOWS were much encreased; tho' at half past II, they were *more* than double in Length to the Height of each Object.

The

The Country beyond the Rivulet began to difclofe itfelf: but was quite *new*.

The Trees woud therefore fpread a SHADE *acrofs* the Road.

The TOPS of the *Houfes* likewife, being Part of them in the Shade; and either *thatched* with Straw, or covered with Slates of a *dufky* Hue; woud prevent their *throwing off* any *ftriking* Colour.

Poffibly the *Encreafe* of Shade *alone*, might give the Face of the Country *below*, a *dark-green* Caft.

It is certain that the Height of the Balloon muft have been very great, to prevent the Sight of public and *Turnpike-Roads*, *above* which it *frequently* paffed, and which had been PLAINLY feen *before* the *Re-afcent*.

For fuppofe the Road but 5 Yards wide, which is lefs than the Truth; if it be allowed that an Object may be diftinguifhed by a *fharp*-fighted Perfon, when its *Diftance* from the Eye does not *exceed* 5156 Times the Diameter of the Object; i. e. when the Object does not fubtend a *lefs* Angle at the Eye than 30 *Seconds* of a Circle, (Smith's Optics, Article 97) which is the *fmalleft* vifible Point, and equal to the 8000th Part of an Inch on the *Retina*;—by multiplying 5 Yards, viz. the Diameter of the public Road, into 5156 (or, in round Numbers, into 5000) Times its Diftance from the Eye in the Balloon; the Product is 25000 Yards: which Product being divided by 1760, the Number of Yards in a Mile, amounts to 14 Miles, and 360 Yards.

Suppofing farther, that a *common* Eye can *only* fee an Object at *half* that Diftance; the Height woud *then* be 7 Miles.

The *Improbability*, therefore, (on Account of the

WELL KNOWN WHEN BELOW. 147

new to him at that *Altitude*, and feemed as if almoft covered with Wood.

176. His *Watch* fhewed the Time of the Day, and the Sun alone *fufficiently* indicated the Point of the Compafs.

The *white* Flag manifefted *no* Change in the Wind.

But whether he was near Liverpool, Wigan, or Manchefter, he coud not difcover.

177. He was entirely LOST in the *blue* *Fields* of Air ; far above the Summits of the Clouds ; tho' the Balloon was in Sight of the Earth, and of Numbers who were gazing at it.

<small>The Country *below* unknown to the Aironaut, *when* in the Balloon.</small>

178. The *Colour* of the new Rivulet was full as RED, as any he had feen before.

He thought it might be an infignificant

the *Warmth* of the Air at that Height, viz. 60°;) of having *foared* to fo great an Altitude, feems to point out, that the SHADOWS muft have contributed a *principal* Share, in preventing a Sight of the public and *Turnpike* Roads.

ficant Brook, which tho' curiously curved, was too small to be inserted in the Map.

Still he continued over it: turning and returning *gently* in small Curves.

179. He presently passed *Northward* of the Rivulet *over* a woody Country, in which he coud discover *no* Variety of *Colouring* either in the Ground Work or Enclosures; the whole having a *dark green* Cast.

Unusual Objects below.
An Appearance of a very distant and remote *Plain* then presented itself; the Size of a moderate Carpet: of a *ruddy* Colour; and surrounded by a *green* Border. Being an unusual Object it continued to engage his Attention.

180. Not far from the first, another of the same Kind, of a more dusky Cast, but *less* and somewhat nearer, that is *more under* him, then attracted his Notice.

He wished to *decipher them*, but in vain.

181. The

181. The Sun shone BRIGHT on both: and in a very few Minutes, the *circular* Prospects *encreased*: which was now become a *regular* and undeniable Signal that the Balloon had begun to *descend*. (Section 17.)

The Prospects opened, which demonstrated his Descent, owing to the Loss of Gass.

The *latter* Plain appeared, at the first, about the Size of a common *Handkerchief*.

The Balloon continued to descend.

182. In a Couple of Minutes, the Plain appeared intersected CLOSELY every Way, like the *Coat* of a *ripening Melon*. Descending a little *lower*; it seemed covered with a *Net*, the *Meshes* of which were distinct. And *lower* still; it extended itself *greatly* on *all* Sides: (at which Time a certain Degree of *Chilliness* prevailed:) and was then *again mistaken*, and looked upon as a DRY *Heath*, deeply overrun with Shrubs of the same Name.

The same Spot perpetually varying to the Eye of the Aironaut.

183. The Descent of the Balloon being *rather* quicker than was expected, or desired; it was deemed expedient

Ballast thrown ou gradually.

dient to have Recourse to the *last* Bag of Sand, which lay open, and weighed 20 Pounds.

It was accordingly thrown out, a Handful at a Time.

The remaining Ballast thrown out at once, in all 20lb. weight. But that Method not seeming *sufficient* to *check* the Descent, when at the Height of 150 or 200 Yards; *all* the Sand was poured out, and the Bag thrown down.

Gentle Landing of the Balloon. This had the desired Effect: and the Balloon continuing to descend with a Motion *uniformly retarded*, alighted, as the DOWN *of a Thistle*, in the gentlest Manner, without ANY *Rebound*.

Anchor and Cable not made use of. 184. There being scarcely a *Breath* of Air abroad, the Aironaut made no Use of his Anchor and Cable: but continued as from the first, STANDING *upright* in the Car; which, having moved a Yard or two *only* along the Ground, rested in a perpendicular Situation.

The Balloon, suspended over him like

like a *vaſt* Umbrella, LEVITATED *vertically* in the grandeſt Manner.

185. He was *alone* when he alighed: but, in a *few* Minutes, found himſelf ſurrounded by the Country-People, who had waded *above Ancle-deep*, and came running from all Parts, to ſee the WONDER, and contribute their *Aſſiſtance*.

186. He *landed* exactly, at 7 Minutes before IV: Thermometer 59: but WHERE he coud *not* tell.

Landed at 53 Minutes paſt III. Thermometer 59.

The firſt Queſtion was " Pray where am I?" And the Anſwer;— in *Lancaſhire*.

On aſking the neareſt Diſtance to a Turnpike-Road; the People ſaid he was within *two Fields* of one, and offered to conduct him thither.

He accepted their Offer, and ſhared *his Liquor* among them.

CHAP-

CHAPTER XXXIII.

Section 187. THE Balloon alighted *near* the *Middle* of a MOSS; called RIXTON-MOSS, a Place he had never before heard of.

Rixton-Moſs, its Magnitude.

It was a large Tract of uncloſed WET Land, above four Miles long and above two broad, interſected by Ditches or Water Courſes, which divide the Moſs into Fields of a *moderate* Size. The whole is ſurrounded by *tall* Foreſt Trees.

This was the *leſſer* of the two duſky Plains, which appeared about the Size of a Handkerchief, and which he wiſhed to decipher, but in vain.

188. Rixton-Moſs is ſituated five Miles North North Eaſt of Warrington, and a little to the left of the Turnpike Road leading from thence to Mancheſter, and 25 from Cheſter.

189. He has ſince been informed that the other Plain, about the Size of

of a moderate *Carpet*, was no *less* a Place than CHAT MOSS, a vast *Tract* of barren *wet* Land, *many* Miles in Extent.

<small>Chat-Moss in Lancashire.</small>

190. Curiosity tempted him to make particular Enquiry concerning the Rivulet over which he hung, *admiring* the Beauty of its serpentine Meanders; and, from a Description given of his Manouvres over *Lymm*, situated to the East of Warrington, and from a peculiar Curve, appearing in the Form of a *true Lover's Knot*, when over the Gunpowder Water-Mills, he was convinced the *Rivulet* coud have been no *other* than the broad Branch of the River MERSEY.

<small>The *Rivulet* seen when *above*, was the River Mersey near Warrington.</small>

191. The AERIAL EXCURSION was performed in two Hours, and a Quarter, within two Minutes.

<small>The Excursion performed in two Hours and a Quarter.</small>

The Distance of the Balloon-Course, if traced along the Ground, 30 Miles. Section 130. (*a*)

192. In comparing the Dates at Bellair and Rixton-Moss; it is certain that

END OF THE RE-ASCENT.

Balloon, unknown to the Aironant, going at the Rate of 30 Miles an Hour.

that the Balloon, excluding the Force of *Ascent*, must have moved *forwards*, during some Part of the Re-ascent, at least at the Rate of 30 Miles an Hour: tho' the Aironaut, for the most Part, imagined he was gliding throu' a serene Atmosphere.

Probably the progressive Motion was encreased, from the Time the unusual Sound was heard, in Section 162.

Note: The Print, representing a CHROMATIC View above the *Level* of the Clouds, of the Country from *Chester* to *Rixton Moss*, is to front the *left* Page, at the End of this Chapter.

END OF THE RE-ASCENT.

CHAPTER XXXIV.

THE SEQUEL.

Flights with the Balloon for THREE Hours longer.

Section 193. THE Sequel contains an Account of *several Flights* made, in Presence of the

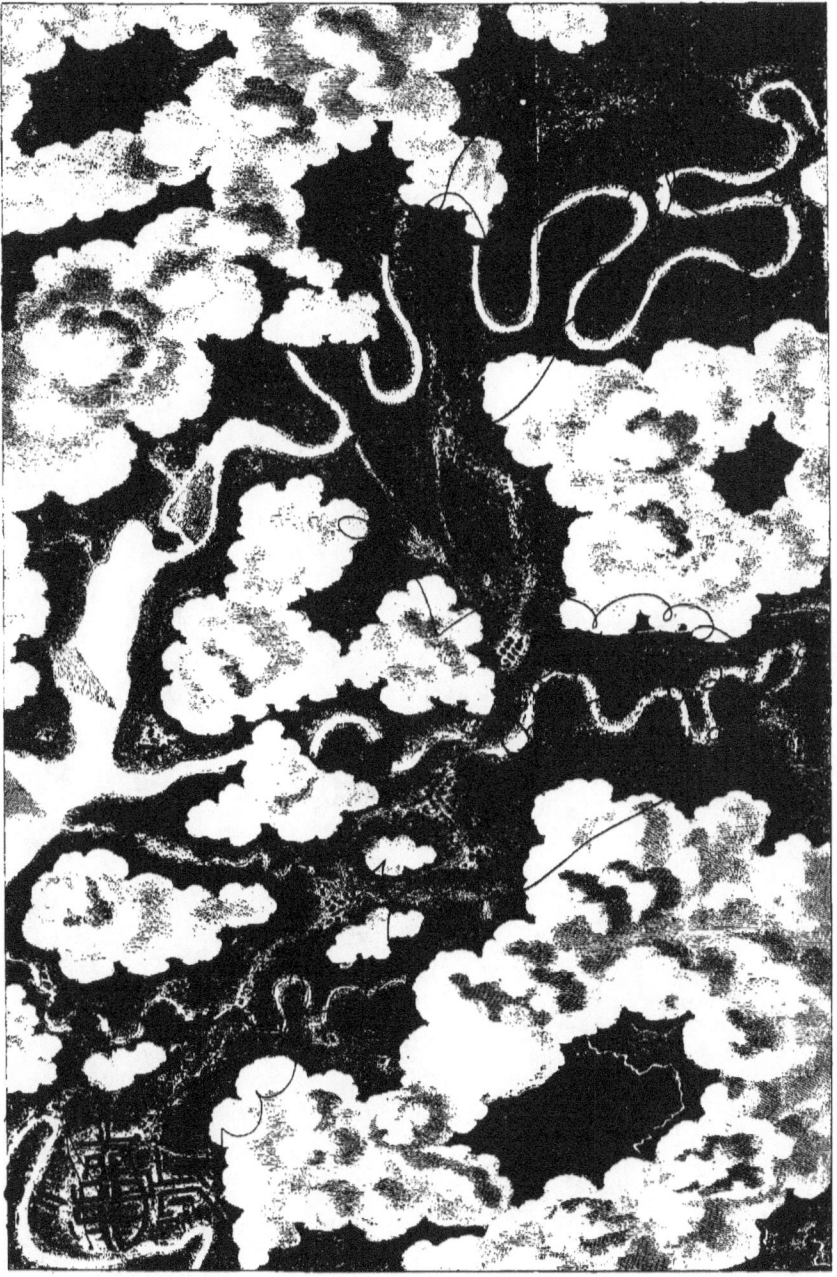

15

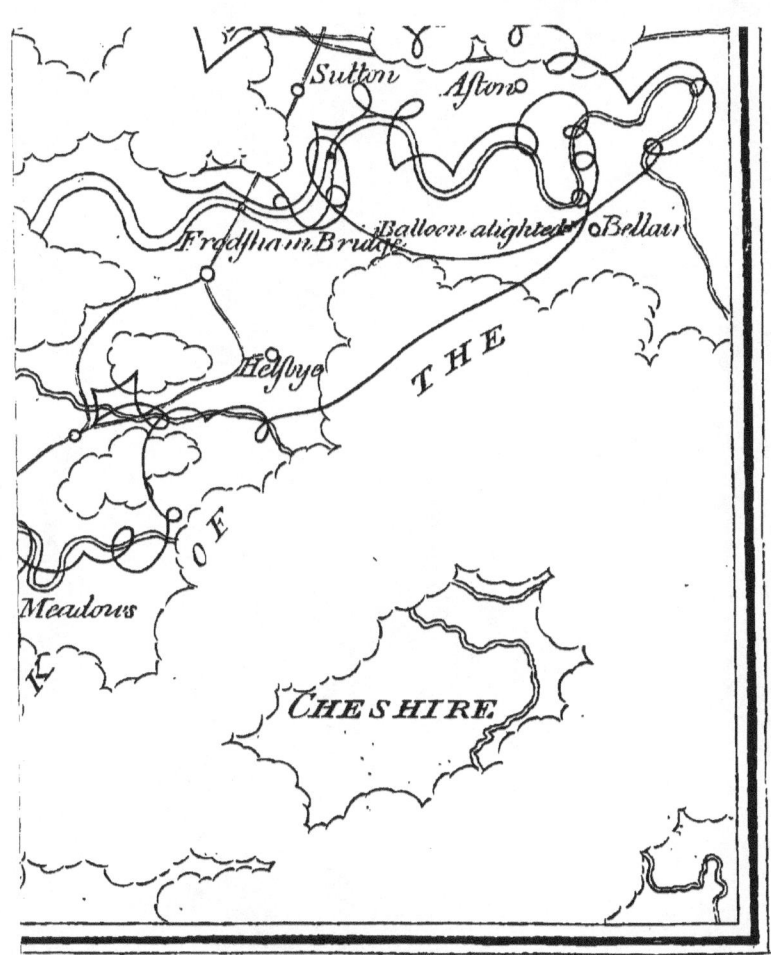

EXPLANATORY Print.   see Page 1111. d.

To be placed at Page 150 of Aëropaidia.

Chap. M.

The **EXPLANATORY** Print. *see Page 111 d.*

the Aironaut, by different Perſons, during *three* Hours, in the Car of the Balloon, viz. from the Time he alighted, till *after* SUNSET.

Rixton-Moſs, LANCASHIRE, IV. o'Clock P. M.

The Afternoon being *fine*, the Sun *bright*, and the Air *calm*; finding the Country People remarkably civilized and kind; and having diſpatched a Meſſenger on Foot to return in a Poſt Chaiſe from Warrington; the Aironaut was reſolved to gratify the Curioſity of his numerous Followers, and give the young People a Taſte for Balloons, by treating them ſucceſſively with an Airing.

194. Indeed it was no inconvenient Method of removing and conducting the Machine: and *poſſibly* different Poſitions of the Balloon might furniſh a *uſeful* Hint.

Having aſked aloud *who choſe to ride,* ſeveral anſwered in the Affirmative. So having pitched upon a young Fellow

The Aironaut indulged the People of the Country with Flights in the Balloon.

low of less Weight than himself; bid him get up, between the Cords, over the Hoop, into the Car; stand near the Middle, and hold an opposite Cord in each Hand.

He obeyed with the greatest Alacrity: and seemed to be *a noisy bold* Adventurer.

The Aironaut first quitted the Car; but continued to conduct the Balloon.

195. The *Aironaut* then got out; and having suffered the Balloon to rise; fastened the End of the Cable to *central* Meshes of the Net, at the Bottom of the Car: ordering the strongest and tallest Man to hold the Cable, and let it go by Degrees till the Anchor or grappling Iron *alone* remained in his Hand.

Behaviour of different Adventurers.

The Balloon now rising *above* the Height of the Trees, and giving the Adventurer a new and extensive Prospect of the Country; he became *silent*; *pale*; his *Countenance* the *Picture* of *Distress*; looking *down* as if for *Help*.

The

The Conductor repeatedly bid him take Courage. But, in vain.

By lowering the Car *within* the Height of the Trees, he seemed to *recover* from his *Dismay*.

CHAPTER XXXV.

Section 196. THE Route of the Balloon being now throu' a *flat woody* Country, with *tall* Trees growing in the Hedge Rows; a Difficulty occurred, how to conduct the Cable, when the Balloon was *above* or *between* the Trees, without entangling: which gave the Conductor much Trouble, as he was frequently obliged to walk round a Field, the Balloon being held in the Center, before he coud espy a proper Opening.

The Procession marched slowly forward: and the young Man was carried

carried among *his Peers* in Triumph through the Air, acrofs the Turnpike-Road, into the Middle of an open Grafs Field, where he defcended; took a Companion *lefs heavy*, and left the Car.

This Stripling was a good Deal furprifed the Inftant he rofe above the Trees; but ventured to look around: and appeared on the *whole* much delighted.

197. A great Concourfe of People were now collected.

Accidental Carriages halted: joined the Cavalcade, and partook of the Diverfion: the *greater* Part following the Balloon throu' the *open* Fields adjoining the Road.

<small>Caution to prevent the Efcape of the Balloon.</small> The Conductor *generally* preferring the beaten Track; yet *fufpecting* the Balloon with its Adventurer in the Car, might *defignedly* be fuffered to *efcape*, took the Precaution to have the Grapple held by *neareft* Relations to the Perfon in the Car.

198. The

198. The Gafs evaporating; a fmart young Fellow, who feemed ready for the Jaunt, ftepped in: on which the former refigned his Place. But he was no fooner raifed a few Yards above his Companions, than the *florid* Colour forfook his Cheeks; he *trembled*; bent himfelf *double* with Fright; and the Balloon was obliged to be hauled down.

199. A fond Mother then requefted that her Child, a fine blooming Girl, might afcend: boafting of her Courage, and comparing it with that of the Perfon who had none.

<small>A Venus in the Car of the Balloon.</small>

The *Venus* fmiled, and mounted her Car with great Spirit.

200. Some Ladies and Gentlemen of the Neighbourhood who had watched the Balloon, while it hung at an immenfe Height over Lymm, and the Gunpowder Works on the River Merfey, came, in their Evening Walk, to meet it: joined the Proceffion; gave the Aironaut *polite* Invitations to

<small>Politenefs of the neighbouring Gentlemen.</small>

to their Houses, and shewed him every possible Civility.

Effect of Air in Motion on the Surface of the Balloon.

201. The Resistance made by the Surface of the Balloon, against the *least Breath* of Air moving *horizontally*, was *frequently* tried by occasionally holding the Grapple: and it was a decided Point, that the *least Motion of the Air* was sufficient, together with the Action of *Levitation*, to prevent the Person, who held the Grapple when the Cable was extended, from transporting the Balloon against the Current: nay it was with Difficulty he coud remain in the *same* Place: the Balloon sometimes pulling him forwards, and almost off his Feet.

Effect of calm Air on the Surface of the Balloon.

202. When the Air was perfectly *calm*, which frequently happened while the Balloon migrated with different Passengers, as the Evening was the finest in the World, and the Country flat and woody in the HedgeRows; it was with *Difficulty* that the Conductor coud draw the Balloon after

after him, faster than the Rate of a moderate *Walk*: viz. three Miles an Hour.

CHAPTER XXXVI.

Section 203. THE Sun set at 34 Minutes past VI. and, tho' it was *then* near that Time, the Post-Chaise was *not* arrived.

<small>Sun set at 34 Minutes past VI.</small>

204. On Enquiry for a dry smooth Meadow, he was recommended to proceed a little farther, to a Place on the Road within three Miles of Warrington.

205. Having by this Time gratified the Curiosity of the Country in admitting Boys and Girls to the Age of six or seven Years, into the Car; and being arrived after Sun-set at the Place appointed, viz. *Milton's Croft-Green*; he ordered the Balloon to be laid on

Y   its

its Side along the Ground: having removed the Car, and opened the Mouth; the inflammable Air or Gafs, was foon preffed out by Means of a *long Pole* rolled *acrofs* it by two Men, ftanding one at each End of the Pole: beginning at the Top or upper Valve, which was held down clofe to the Ground; and ending at the Mouth or Neck.

It was then rolled up, put into the Car; and the whole Apparatus placed on the Top of the Chaife which arrived the Moment wanted.

Balloon put up at 53 Minutes paft VI.

206. The Operation was completed at 53 Minutes paft VI: the Conductor having accompanied the Balloon on Foot exactly THREE Hours.

Balloon in the Air five Hours and a Quarter.

207. The Balloon had therefore continued *floating* in the Air, with different Perfons, in the whole, for the Space of five Hours and a Quarter.

The Conductor, promifing to accept

cept the very polite Invitation offered him by Mr. *Stanton*, a Gentleman who is principally concerned in the Gunpowder-Works upon the Merfey; called at his Houfe, and partook of fome Refrefhments.

He then drove to Warrington, where he was met by a Perfon whom Curiofity had infpired to follow the Balloon *on Foot* from Chefter, as long as he coud keep it *in View*.

208. Mr. Lunardi likewife with great Civility difpatched his Servant to affift the Aironaut in *the Care* of the Balloon; but he did not arrive in Time; not reaching Warrington till VIII. at Night: having loft Sight of the Balloon about *Darefbury*, four Miles from Warrington.

209. Nor was it vifible to any, at leaft very few, of the Inhabitants of that Town, which was equally hidden from the Aironaut: who, *then* ignorant of his Situation, muft have
remained

remained a confiderable Time fufpended above the Clouds; which concealed both the Town and River.

He faw Warrington but twice when ABOVE: for a fhort Time, at a great Diftance, and a *mediate* Altitude.

210. The following Day he returned to Chefter: was met by the Militia-Mufic, and ufhered with loud Huzzaes into his native City.

On his fafe Arrival; befides the private and fincere Congratulations of his Relations and Friends; the Bells rang: his Flags were carried in Proceffion, and every public Demonftration of Joy was fhewn on the Occafion.

TO THE INHABITANTS OF CHESTER

T H A N K S.

END OF THE EXCURSION
THROU' THE AIR.

(165)

AIROPAIDIA.

CHAPTER XXXVII.

OBSERVATIONS, HINTS, AND CONJECTURES, ON THE SUBJECT OF THE BALLOON AND EXCURSION FROM CHESTER THE EIGHTH OF SEPT. 1785.

OF THE WEATHER, IN THE VICINITY OF CHESTER, ABOUT THE TIME OF THE EXCURSION.

Section 211. FOR more than ten Days *before* the Balloon-Voyage, the Wind had blown (*interruptedly* on Account of the Sea-Breeze) from South and South by West.

Monday the 5th of September:

A Conjunction of the Planet Mercury and the Moon, at ONE in the Afternoon.

Tuesday the 6th:

A violent Hurricane in the South of England, as London, Portsmouth, &c.

The

The same Day at Chester North-North-West, and distant from London 182 Miles; South-Breeze; Rain most of the Day. Thermometer at Noon in the Shade, 62: and 14 Divisions colder each Night, than the *following* Day, at an Average of five Years. Barometer, below *Much Rain*, viz. at 28 Inches $\frac{9}{10}$ths.

Wednesday the 7th:

Violent Squalls from South and South-West, with hazy Air, till half past IV in the Afternoon. Thermom. 58; Barom. Changeable, viz. $29\frac{1}{2}$.

Thursday the 8th, which was the Day of the Excursion:

Much bright Sun. (On Enquiry) calm *below* till half past III in the Afternoon, then West Sea-Breeze: South-West Breeze *above* till half past IV. Calm bright Evening.

Also the upper Stratum of Clouds thin and *white*, in *quick* Motion, when seen from *below* till Noon: at which Time the Sky was almost cloudless: and, from *above* the upper Stratum, were seen, interspersed, Multitudes of detached Thunder-Clouds in large Masses, rising at Intervals, in the *Middle* of the upper Surfaces of white Clouds, and stretching *above* them.

Friday and Saturday moderate: South and South-West Breeze.

Sunday the 11th. The Planet Mercury stationary.

Cloudy Morn. South-West Breeze. Thermom. at 60 at Noon. Barom. *above*, Changeable, viz. at $29\frac{1}{2}$. MUCH THUNDER and Rain in the Afternoon.

212. Quere,

ABOUT THE TIME OF THE EXCURSION.   167

212. Quere, Had the *Thunder*-Clouds on Thurſday, tho' not remarked by any from BELOW, yet viſible to a great Extent from the Balloon *above* them,—any Connexion with the *Thunder* that happened THREE Days after?

Anſwer: It appears to the Obſerver, that the Thunder was *gradually* collecting in the Air from Thurſday till Sunday: and if ſo; will not Balloons, when more *frequent*, prognoſticate the Weather, *by Sight*, better than any other known Methods? Weather, to be prognoſticated, *by Sight*, from the Balloon

---

CHAPTER XXXVIII.

ON CERTAIN APPEARANCES AT DIFFERENT ALTITUDES OF THE BALLOON.

Section 213. THE higheſt viſible *white* Clouds, often ſeen in detached Streaks, during the fineſt and alſo in the worſt Weather, (if not intercepted by lower Clouds) and which, when melting away, are known in ſome Counties by the common Appellation of Horſe-Tails; and, ſuſpended over Great-Britain, are frequently *marbled* or dappled by the Wind; putting on the Appearance of white Waves, like Sea-Sands ruffled and left by a rapid Tide;—had been diſturbed, ſeparated, and almoſt *melted* down by the *Storm* the Day preceding the Excurſion. Of the higheſt viſible Clouds which are always *white*.

Two of them *only* were ſtill viſible in Streaks, near the Sun's Place, at the firſt Aſcent. They ſeemed

seemed without Motion, and became afterwards *invisible*.

Sauſſure, the celebrated Profeſſor of Philoſophy at Geneva, is very exact in his Definition, Deſcription, and Height of theſe Appearances: and thinks it *probable*, their Situation may be " *at least fifteen Engliſh Miles above the Surface of the Earth.*"

" Car quand je conſidere ces fines Pommelures, &c." " For when I conſider theſe delicate Dapplings, which, in a Series of fair Weather, begin to cover the azure Vault of Heaven with a white and tranſparent Gauze, and which portend Rain a long Time before it happens; I am led to believe they occupy a very elevated Situation in the Atmoſphere." (Eſſais ſur l'Hygrometrie, P. 271.)

It ſeems however that *Croſbie*, in his Excurſion from Dublin on the 25th of January 1785, pierced throu' and ſoared above theſe *fine Webs*, at the Height of 16 Inches by the Barometer in a *froſty* Air.

Of the Chilliness perceived at a certain Height.

214. It has been already noted, that at a certain Height, a Kind of CHILLINESS was perceived, not aſcertainable by the Thermometer.

The Senſation was *ſuddenly* impreſſed four Times, in aſcending and deſcending to and from the ſame Height, viz. about 26 and 27 Inches, equivalent to between 500 and 1000 Yards above the Surface of the Earth at the firſt Aſcent.

From the Uniformity of Effect at the ſame Height; the Senſation may be aſcribed to the ſame Cauſe, viz. the Level of the firſt or lower Tier of Clouds: altho' the Aironaut did not paſs pafs throu' any visible Cloud or Vapour, during the Excursion. See Section 93.

215. At the same Height likewise, tho' the Observations have not been set down at large; the Appearances of the Earth and Clouds were very remarkable. *Remarkable Appearances of Earth and Clouds.*

During the Ascent of the Balloon, between the Altitudes of 26 and 27 Inches; the *circular* Prospects of the subjacent Earth *instantly* contracted, and, during the Descent, about the same Height, *instantly* enlarged themselves to the Eye of the Aironaut.

216. At the same Height mentioned before, the *circular* Prospects of the Clouds appeared on the same horizontal Plane with the Eye: tho' at the Distance of a Mile. See Section 49.

In *this* Situation, the Observer endeavoured to discover the Thickness of the *Stratum* of Clouds: but was always baffled by a Deception of Sight worth recording.

The *Strata* were plainly composed of three or more Heights of Clouds, *sailing* at great Intervals, one above the other: all which regularly *vanished*, as he approached their respective Levels: as if *instantly* thrown into the Circumference of a Circle, whose Radius was a Mile.

During the Ascent, in passing their supposed Level, the Clouds *instantly* appeared *far below* him: and during the Descent, as far *above*.

217. Quere: Is it not from the same Cause, that all Vapour is *generally* invisible to a certain Height and Distance from the Eye?

It being incontrovertible that more Vapours rise about NOON, than at any other Hour, particularly

cularly at Sea, while the Sun continues to *shine*: which, notwithstanding, are wholly *invisible*, till arrived at a *certain* Height?

Visibility of Vapours by mere Distance.

And hence the Visibility of Vapours by *mere* Distance, which contains a sufficient Number of Particles to intercept and refract the Light, without Cold, Condensation, or *actual* Accumulation: viz. by Refrangibility of those primary Rays of Light, which Air and Vapour united are most *apt* to reflect or transmit.

Monsf. Saussure has proved by his Horse-Hair compàrable Hygrometer, that " the Air shews Signs of *greatest* Humidity an Hour after Sunrise, and of *least* Humidity, between three and four in the *Afternoon*." But the Air being *then* also the hottest, will *dissolve* or evaporate the greatest Quantity of Vapours, and raise them *above* the Hygrometer (which by its *Heat* will not retain, but on the contrary repel and *dissipate* them) to great Heights in the Atmosphere.

See " Essais sur l'Hygrometrie, C. 6, P. 315."

218. In general then:

Is not the *Cause* of the above Deceptions, *not* an *Absence*, but a *Transparency of Vapour* to a certain Distance: (just as the Zenith *appears* CLOUDLESS, when the Air is *overcast* around;) beyond which Distance, the *Number* and relative Proximity of Particles with Respect to the Eye, is such, as to intercept the Rays of Light: *when only*, they put on the *Colour* of Air, and Form of Vapour and Cloud?

And hence the probable Reason, why NO *circular* Horizon of the Earth's Surface was presented during the Excursion, Section 79: and why

why it seldom has or can present itself to Aironauts or *Mountaineers*, at any *considerable* Height above the Region or Level of Clouds, even tho' Clouds do *not* appear in the Air, either to themselves, or to Spectators *below*.

This Point seems capable of Illustration by Analogy, from the Impossibility of encreasing the *Magnitude*, and at the same Time, *Distinctness* of distant Objects, seen throu' a *common* Telescope; on Account of the Quantity of Vapours between them and the Eye   Which VAPOURS may be magnified till the Object appears confused and obscure; and even at last become substituted in the Place of the Object, under the Form of Opacity and *Cloudiness*.

219. The *greater* the Height of the Balloon, the more *contracted* was the Circle of Vapour below it; and the more limited the Prospect of the Earth's Surface below the Vapour.

220. It seemed probable that the Sun shone as *bright* on the Countries around the Observer, as on Objects immediately below him: which Objects coud not have been illuminated by the Sun's Rays, darting throu' the APPARENT and *contracted* OPENING under him; as the Rays which shone on the Balloon, fell beyond the *Opening*, *obliquely* on Clouds which caught the Shadow of the Balloon.

221. The extreme *Rarity* or *Tenuity* of the Vapours was *evident* from the *progressive* Course of the Balloon, which was *always* in the Center of a *circular* Opening, limiting the lower Prospects; except when the Spectator lost all Sight

of the Earth, by dense, watry, intervening Clouds.

Novel Situation peculiar to the Balloon, again described.

This *august* central Situation, ALWAYS CHANGING YET STILL THE SAME, had the most striking Effect on the Senses and Imagination. Yet, however pleasing the Recollection of this GLORIOUS APPEARANCE; however *strongly* impressed, accurately described, or richly painted; it must fall infinitely short of the original SENSATION. Unity and Sameness were there contrasted with *perpetual Variety*: Beauty of Colouring; Minuteness, and consummate Arrangement;—with *Magnificence* and *Splendor: actual* Immensity;—with *apparent* Limitation:—all which were *distinctly* conveyed to the Mind, at the *same* Instant, throu' the Intervention of the Organs of Sight; and, to complete the Scene, was added the Charm of NOVELTY.

CHAPTER XXXIX.

CONJECTURES ON THE CAUSES OF THE CIRCULAR TRANSPARENCY TO A CERTAIN DISTANCE BELOW THE BALLOON, AND OF THE RED LIGHT FROM THE SEA AND RIVERS, WHEN SEEN ABOVE THE LEVEL OF THE SUPERIOR CLOUDS.

On the circular Transparency.

Section 222. QUERE: As Red is the heaviest and Blue the lightest Colour; and as *red* Rays blended at a certain Angle with *blue* Rays, produce Opacity: further; as RED

is

is the *predominant* Colour reflected from Water, while in the Form of *dense* Cloud, for Instance at the Rising and Setting of the Sun; and BLUE the Colour always reflected from the light Medium of Air or Sky; Does not this Mixture of least and most refrangible Rays, which, when aided with the intermediate primary ones, causes a *Transparency* near and round the Eye of a Spectator placed either on Earth or among the Clouds; produce, at a greater Distance and different Angle, such a Degree of Opacity, as actually to give the Idea of Clouds surrounding him at a Distance?

The latter Part at least is true, that Vapour and Air, which are *naturally* qualified to *transmit* RED and BLUE, rather than any other Light, will, at a certain Angle, when *blended*, produce an OPACITY. (See the Letter sent by NEWTON from Cambridge to Dr. Derham, in order to be presented to the Royal Society,—in " Miscellanea Curiosa, Vol. I, Page 109.")

Quere: May not the Rivers below act as a Prism; as Clouds, about Sun-set or Sun-rise, do to a Spectator on Earth, and reflect only the primary Colour RED, the *heaviest* and least refrangible Ray?

On the red Light from the Sea and Rivers.

It being also considered that Refraction cannot change the primary Colour: nor are Rays, in the Direction from below to the Zenith, refracted; tho' seen from a rarer into a denser Medium.

Possibly, a Pencil of Rays, in coming up from the River below may be stripped or drained by the double Absorption of the Atmosphere and River, and the Colour RED only, suffered to reach

reach the Eye: "being the laſt to quit its Baſis the Water." (See Morgan's Obſervations on the Light of Bodies, &c. &c. Phil. Tranſ. for the Year 1785, Part 1, Vol. 75, Chap. 91.)

CHAPTER XXXX.

ON THE EXCESSIVE DIMINUTION OF OBJECTS ON THE SURFACE OF THE EARTH, TO A SPECTATOR SITUATED ABOVE THE REGION OF CLOUD, AT THE BAROMETRIC HEIGHT OF NEAR A MILE AND HALF, PERPENDICULAR.

Recapitulation of the Scenery below.

Section 223. THE Earth's Surface was preſented to the Eye throu' a *circular* Opening as already deſcribed.

This Opening diſcovered a *Plain*, ſmooth and level as a Die: a Sort of *ſhining* Carpet, enriched with an endleſs Variety of Figures depicted *without* Shadow, as on a Map: what was really Shadow forming a ſeparate Colour, and not conſidered at the Time, as *Shadow*. The Objects were diſtinctly marked, and perfectly known to be Miniatures of the Face of Nature.

All was *Colouring*: no Outline: yet each Appearance curiouſly defined by a ſtriking Contraſt of ſimple Colours, which ſerved to diſtinguiſh the reſpective Boundaries with moſt exact Preciſion, and inconceivable Elegance.

RED Rivers, YELLOW Roads, Encloſures YELLOW and *light* GREEN, Woods and Hedges *dark* GREEN, were the only Objects clearly diſtinguiſhable,

MODE OF ESTIMATING DISTANT OBJECTS. 175

tinguishable, and their Colouring extremely vivid. The Sun's Rays reflected from the Surface of the Sea, and other Waters, dazzled the Sight.

ALL living Creatures were invisible.

224. The Area of each Inclosure, computed to contain a certain Number of Acres, was seen from above under the Form of a Miniature Picture of a certain Magnitude or visible Extension, perpetually diminishing, as the Eye recedes to a greater Distance.

And the Case is similar, whether the Miniature be seen from *above,* or *along* the Ground.

The Miniature also lessens as the Distance encreases, according to a certain Proportion so exactly (*a*); That,

1. If the *Distance* and *Magnitude* of a tangible Object be known by Mensuration; a Judgment is formed, and Laws laid down, for its corresponding *Miniature* on the Eye.

2. If the *Miniature* be seen, and *Distance* known by Mensuration; the Mind forms a Judgment of its tangible *Magnitude.*

3. And lastly, if the *Miniature* be seen, and *Magnitude* of a tangible Object is known by Mensuration; the Mind makes an Effort, to the Estimation of its Distance from the Eye.

These

(*a*) The MAGNITUDE of an Object *decreases,* as the SQUARES of its Distance from the Eye *increase.*

At whatever Distance, for Example, the Eye can see any Object clearly; as at the Distance of a Foot, or a Yard, if the Object be removed to *twice* that Distance; it will appear 4 Times smaller than it did before: 2 multiplied into 2, equals 4, which is the Square of 2: in the same Manner, if the Object be removed to thrice the Distance from the Eye; it will appear 9 Times as small, as at the first Distance: for 3 into 3 gives 9, the Square of 3: and so of any farther Distance,

Thefe are fome, among many Modes of Comparifon, by which the Mind acquires a tolerable Degree of Proficiency, in eftimating *Diftances* of familiar Objects, *known* from the Appearance of their refpective Miniatures on the Fund or Bottom of the Eye.

And fo far moft Theories agree.

But fuch *ocular* Teft is only true, while the Comparifon is made in *nearly* the fame Medium.

For an Object, if feen at the fame Diftance *along* the Ground, will appear lefs as it rifes above it; and leaft in the Zenith; as the Sun and Moon, at Setting or Rifing, appear *large and oval*; but at their greateft Elevation, are *fmall* and *round:* becaufe being feen, when paffed out of a Medium impregnated with Vapours, which in fome Meafure intercept the Rays of Light: for the FAINTER (*a*) a diftant Object appears, the *greater* it is appprehended to be. (*b*)

Poffibly indeed an Object at the fame Diftance, if brighter at one Time than another, will *contract the Pupil* in Proportion to its Brightnefs: which may have the fame Effect, as if the Object had made a *fmaller* Miniature on the Retina; and will regularly ftrike the Mind with an Idea of *Magnitude*, *only* equal to its correfponding *Contraction*; i. e. lefs, when the Object is bright, and greater when faint.

225. If a like Reafoning be applied to the Afcent of Balloons; and it be faid that they do not rife
fo

(*a*) See " Berkeley's New Theory of Vifion, Section 67."
(*b*) Dr. Smith having Recourfe to *intervening Objects*; the Writer cannot affent to the Validity of his Argument, illuftrated by a well-known Figure, to folve the Appearance of the *horizontal Moon*. See " Prieftley's Hiftory of Light and Colours, Page 712."

ON THE CAUSES OF THE DIMINUTION.

so high as is imagined, because their Magnitude is diminished, merely from being elevated into a Portion of the Atmosphere *least* impregnated with Vapours; it will follow, that to a Spectator in the Balloon; known Objects on the Surface of the Earth below,—being seen from a rarer into a denser Medium, also into one which contain a great Quantity of Vapours;—shoud appear *larger*, than when seen along the Ground, at a Distance equal to its Height in the Balloon: all which is contrary to Matter of Fact: particularly if the Barometer gives a proper Estimate of the Height, of which there is little Doubt: a proper Allowance being made, *in certain Cases*, on Account of the Refraction: for, as before mentioned, (Section 44.) Objects seen from the Balloon at a Mile and Half *barometric* Height, continued, with invariable Uniformity, to suggest the Idea of at least seven Miles.

226. By a general Comparison of Enclosures, and of separate Buildings when they coud be distinguished from the Balloon above the Region of Cloud, with the most distant Extremities, (on the horizontal Level) of Fields or Houses situated along the Sides of Hills or Mountains, at a known Distance by Miles, making Allowance for their being seen in a straight Line;—the latter seemed at least five Times *larger* than the *former:* supposing them at equal Distances.

To give an Instance. Supposing the most distant Extremities of a known Building or Enclosure, situated on the Side of a Hill or Mountain, presented a Miniature of a *familiar* Magnitude to the Eye of the Spectator on the Ground, at the known Distance of a Mile and Half; the same Object when seen from the Balloon at the same *barometric* Height, appeared full five Times less.

This Comparison was made by Memory, the Morning after the Excursion, tho' suggested while in the Balloon, from the wonderful Minuteness of all Objects then presented to the Eye.

The Author being likewise familiarized to judge of Heights; having been on several of the chief Mountains in Europe: also, of comparative Distances, from his Situation near a large City, in a populous, enclosed Country; on a high Plain, within View of the Sea, Mountains, Hills, Enclosures, Buildings, and Objects whose Magnitude and Distances were known.

227. The Balloon itself, a Globe twenty-five Feet in Diameter, was seen in the Air on the Day of Ascent, at the Distance of 19 Miles.

The Magnitude of Objects seen from the Balloon compared with those of the Sun or Moon near the Meridian, when seen from below.

228. The Reason already given, for the Solution of the famous Question concerning the apparent Magnitude of the horizontal Moon, seems no less applicable to Objects on the Earth's Surface, when seen from the Balloon: which *Diminution* of Objects *below* confirms the Defect of Dr. Smith's Hypothesis.

For, as they appeared *extremely bright*; being shone on by the Sun, and seen throu' the Air in a perpendicular Line, containing the least possible Quantity of Vapour; the Brightness must have exceeded that of the same Objects, when seen along the Ground: and consequently the Miniatures of the former must have been less than the latter, and also their respective Distances *seem greater*.

CHAPTER

CHAPTER XXXXI.

CONJECTURES ON THE CAUSES WHICH INFLUENCE THE DESCENT OF BALLOONS IN THEIR PASSAGE OVER WATER.

1. COnjectures concerning the regular Tendency of the Balloon to *descend* on its *Approach* towards WATER. — Recapitulation of Facts.

2. Its *greatest* Descent, when in the Zenith, over the Middle of Rivers.

3. Recovery and *Re-ascent* to the former Level, as it *recedes* from them.

Section 229. Article 1. On the first Ascent in the Castle-Yard, Chester, the Balloon gently moved towards the River Dee, and the Sea.

And woud probably have gone out to Sea, if the ascensive Power had not presently raised it above the Influence of the Water; into an upper Current of Air, which was visible at that Time, and for two Hours before the Ascent, by the Motion of superior Clouds in a safe Direction towards the Land.

229. 2. The Balloon was *affected* in passing across the River Goway, and Trafford Meadows, which are a Mile wide: first moving Westward, and again towards the Sea; making several Curves: then resting and *lingering* between Great and Little Barrow: as the Aironaut was *well* informed by Persons of *Veracity*, who observed it: his Attention being engaged at that Time by other Objects.

229. 3. A

229. 3. A proportionable Effect was obferved in *croffing* a fmall Brook near Alvanley.

229. 4. The River Wever and its broad Meadows above Frodfham-Bridge actually ftopped the farther Progrefs of the Balloon: tho' its Courfe was *merely* ACROSS the River.

The Deviation was gently tho' *invariably* towards the SEA: and, if not *timely* prevented, the Balloon muft have fallen in the Middle of the Channel.

229. 5. The fame Cafe woud have happened on the Re-afcent at Bellair; if the *levitating* Force had *not* as at firft, overcome the Influence of the WATERS, and lifted the Balloon into the *fame* upper Current, which continued to move in its former fafe Direction.

229. 6. Different Branches of the Duke of Bridgewater's Canal near Prefton-Brook might *poffibly* affect it in a fmall Degree: and, tho' Clouds a little afterwards, fecluded the Aironaut from a Sight of the Earth; yet the Balloon was known to hang, for fome Time, over the Merfey near Warrington.

229. 7. The Balloon defcended and alighted on the Middle of a large Tract of wet Mofs Ground.

The Writer faw Sadler's Balloon rife at Manchefter, the 11th May, 1785, and defcend near Blencow-Bridge, at the Conflux of *two* Rivers.

The above Facts give fufficient Indications of the conftant Tendency which Balloons have, to defcend on Water.

CHAPTER

CHAPTER XXXXII.

Section 230. THREE Causes seem generally to concur in producing the Effect of Descent, over Water.
1. The Water itself.
2. The Air above it.
3. Change of Temperature.

Section 231. Article 1. So long as Gafs escapes from the Balloon; it will be instantly and *reciprocally* attracted, throu' the *Crevices*, by the Moisture contained in the *Air*, particularly over *Rivers*: its specific *Gravity* within the Balloon, woud be encreased, (*a*) and consequently the Balloon itself rendered less buoyant:

The Gafs woud, on the contrary, be repelled by *electric* Air: which woud lessen its Tendency to escape, throu' the Pores of the Silk.

But it is *presumed* that Air-tight Balloons will be little affected by *external* Moisture.

231. 2. Moist Air over Water being generally cooler than over the adjacent Land, will, so long as the Gafs continues at its former Temperature, assist and raise the Balloon *thus* moving into a *denser* Stratum: but no sooner is the Balloon contracted by the external Cold, than it descends into a Medium of Air, whose specific Gravity is proportionable to the contracted Bulk of the Balloon, and rests when equal to it.

231. 3. Water is also a Conductor of Electricity, tho' a feeble one: and there is moreover a
strong

(*a*) Phil. Transf. for 1785, Part 1, Page 287.

ſtrong chemical Affinity between WATER, inflammable Air, Gaſſes, Floguiſton, and Electricity. *(a)*

231. 4. Water will therefore CONDUCT the Gaſs to itſelf: i. e. will draw the Balloon *downwards*, and with accelerating Velocity; as the Attraction is ſtronger, the nearer the Water.

231. 5. But if the Air over the Water be warmer than that over Land; then the Balloon, moving into a warmer Medium, as over the Sea in froſty Weather, moſt undoubtedly deſcends: till the included Gaſs has received the additional Encreaſe of Temperature from that of the Air, at which Time it will have a Tendency to re-aſcend, and will reſt ſuſpended in Equilibrio, as in the former Caſe.

The above Cauſes however may be conſidered as *trivial*.

The firſt may be avoided by making the Balloon *Air-tight*: and the ſecond eaſily guarded againſt by throwing out a little *Ballaſt*.

The *only* formidable one, if any, is

THE DEPRESSION OF THE ATMOSPHERE.

This it will be neceſſary to conſider with ſome Degree of Attention.

CHAPTER

(a) Cavallo's Treatiſe on Air, Page 576. Vitriolic Acid Air, Alkaline Air, and other elaſtic Fluids, are inſtantly ABSORBED by *Water*; (Page 673.) Inflammable Air, and fixed Air, are likewiſe ABSORBED by WATER. (Page 434)

CHAPTER XXXXIII.

Section 232. WHOEVER consults Antiquity, *(a)* or is acquainted with modern Mèteorism, will ascent to the Truth of the Facts there recited, viz. That the Storms of DISPERSION called *Prester-John*, and *Ox-Eye* over Table Bay at the Cape of Good-Hope (not to mention those of COLLECTION, as *Whirlwinds*(*b*) and *Waterspouts*;) *descend* on Sea and Land from the *middle* Regions of the Air, often *perpendicularly* DOWNWARDS : and then blow violently from a Center, TO all Parts of the Compass at once : a necessary Consequence of their beating *forcibly* upon the Land or Water.

The Ancients maintained that the Origin of Wind was a mere *Depression* and *Percussion* from the Cold of the middle *Region :* and it shoud be remarked that their Observations were made on the *Continent*, and in *warm* Climates.

Now what is seen to Excess in the *hottest* and
coldest

(*a*) Nam fit, ut interdum tanquam demissâ Columnâ
 In Mare de Cœlo descendat.—Lucr. L. 6. V. 425.
Una Eurus Notusque ruunt, creberque Procellis
Africus. Also
Omnia Ventorum *concurrere* Prælia vidi. VIRGIL.

(*b*) Franklin's Account of Whirlwinds and Waterspouts, in his Miscellaneous Tracts. Lowthorp's Abridgement of Phil. Transf. Vol. 2. Page 103. Varenius Geogr. Gen. C. 21. Pag. 265. A clear Account of the Effects of a DEPRESSION is to be met with in " the History of Jamaica, in 3 vols. vol. 3. Page 800. on *Trade and Land Winds.*"

coldest Climates; (*a*) most probably takes Place, in a less Degree, in temperate ones.

Therefore, on a Change of Weather, the upper Atmosphere *descends:* whether its Effects are *Cold*, as in Winter; *Warmth*, as in Spring; *Wind* or *Wet*; at the proper Seasons of the Year.

233. The Balloon, with which Dicker Junior ascended at Bristol, April 19, 1784, on a WINDY Day, proved the Truth of the Conjecture: for tho' the Aironaut threw out most of his Ballast; yet after each Ascent and Recovery, he was repeatedly darted *downwards* EVEN with the Ground (*b*).

234. A similar Event happened to Crosbie, in his Passage over the Sea from Dublin to England; for, tho' he too discharged his Ballast, the Wind kept him *down* and EVEN with the Water.

The Weather at that Time seems to have been an Εxνέφιας, Procella, Percussion, Squall, or Tornado, i. e. a Storm of DEPRESSION, and DISPERSION.

235. The Eknèfiai Winds come from cool Points on each Side the North.

Bacon also observes that all BOISTEROUS Winds,

(*a*) Monf. Maupertius has found, that the extreme Cold at Tornea, in the northern Regions beyond the Artic Circle, came directly from *above*: see "La Figure de la Terre," Page 59. Il semble que le vent souffle—de tous Côtés à la Fois: et il lance la *Neige* avec une telle Impetuosité, qu'en un Moment tous les Chemins sont perdus. "It seems that the Wind blows from all Points of the Compass at once," &c.

(*b*) The Doctrine of smokey Chimnies distinctly treated of under the Article SMOKE, in the Encyclopædia Britannica, may receive some Improvement, from Circumstances which ascertain the sudden Descent, Elevation, and quick Depression of *Columns* or rather *Torrents* of Air, viz. by widening the Tubes, and covering their Tops.

Winds, as *Procella*, *Typho*, and *Turbo*, have the evident Direction of a Precipice, or Projection *downwards*, more than other Winds: they seem to rush down like a Torrent or Cascade: and are then reverberated or beat back from the Earth, in all Directions.

Stubble, Corn, or Hay in the Meadows are raised, and spread around in the Form of an EXTENDED CANOPY, *(inverted Cone, elliptic Solid,* and *hyperbolic Curve.)* See " Bacon's Historia Ventorum, Pag. 43, ad Articulum 10. (*a*)

236. If then it be allowed to reason from that Analogy which took Place in most of the Cases already mentioned; the *gentler* Depression of Balloons over Water in *milder* Weather, may be owing to a Cause somewhat similar, tho' not so evidently an immediate Object of the Senses, viz. *an actual tho' invisible Descent of Air upon the Water.*

237. Blanchard in his Passage over the Sea from Dover to Bologne in France, when near the Middle of the Channel, suffered an unexpected Depression; and at the same Time was nearly BECALMED.

A CALM also took Place on the Irish Sea: which must have prevented Crosbie from landing,—without *Wings*, or some *propulsive* Machinery, connected with the Balloon.

238. Lunardi

(a) It is thought more *candid*, and will to *many* be more *satisfactory*; to make occasional References to different Authors who have treated distinctly on a Subject, and leave the Reader to draw his own Conclusions by applying to their *express* Words;—than, either to insert abundant Quotations; or *weave* their Thoughts into the *Texture* of the Work: which must encrease its Bulk, without producing any Thing either new or instructive.

238. Lunardi rose from Liverpool when the Wind blew *boisterously*: yet was *becalmed* twenty Minutes over the *broad* Turn of the Mersey near Ince, when above the Level of the Wind: and, descending into the same Stream of Wind, was hurried along towards Beeston-Castle in Cheshire.

CHAPTER XXXXIV.

Depressing Columns of Air known to the Egyptians. Section 239. THE Existence of depressing Columns of Air was well known to a People more ancient than either Romans or Greeks.

240. The sultry Climate of Egypt, whose Situation is that of an extensive Meadow watered by a *broad* River, and enclosed by Mountains to the East and West; consequently not subject to general horizontal Currents of Air, except along the Line of its Meridian,—is *the Country*, wherein Columns of COOL Air descending on the Water, woud be soon observed.

And they, in Fact, were almost the only People who applied the Observation to common Life: having, according to Herodotus, as well as later Writers, built lofty Structures OPEN AT THE TOP. By which Means the cool Air RUSHING downwards greatly refreshed the Inhabitants.

The ancient Pantheon, at present called All Saints Church, now standing at Rome; built in the lowest Situation of a Street named the Piazza di Navona is on this Construction: and the Hint probably taken from an Egyptian Model.

241. In all inland Countries, whose Lakes are

are frequently surrounded by Mountains, as Bala-Pool in North-Wales; those of Westmoreland and Cumberland; the Lake of Geneva in Swisserland;—the Air rushes FORCIBLY on the Surface of the Water in descending Torrents: this the Writer has frequently observed. (*a*)

(In other Languages, the Words applicable to Wind on a Lake, or the Ocean, signify Descent: as, Καταβαινω, and Επικειμαι· also the Northerly or *descending* Wind corresponded to the Εκνεφιας· while the Southerly or *ascending* Wind answered to the Απογη.)

All this, which may be allowed to take Place in *bad* Weather, may perhaps be excepted to, in *fine*, and still more so, in the *finest* Weather.

As the slightest Change is first observable on the Surface of Water, whether on Lakes or the Ocean, the *Descent of Air* in the finest Weather is familiar to Mariners by the Appellation of LIGHT AIRS, playing in Eddies: and particularly in the *variable* Latitudes; i. e. between 32 and 42: to these the Writer can also witness: as well as on small and large inland Lakes, by partial *Dimplings and Rufflings* of the Surface.

OBJECTION TO THE THEORY REMOVED.

242. It may be objected to the above Theory, that the Wind plainly blows in an horizontal Direction, as may be seen from the Motion of Clouds and Trees.

(*a*) Once, particularly, in the Month of January, at Lausanne: Farenheit's Thermometer at 7 only: the Country covered with Snow; and a North Wind beating VIOLENTLY on the Lake, which continued liquid without Ice: owing, perhaps, in *Part*, to subterranean Heat, and Exhalations.

To which it may be anfwered, that if Clouds are not befide the Queftion; as it is not afferted that a fingle Column of Air prefles from fo great a Height to the Earth; (tho' it be the Cafe in Squalls;) yet it is extremely difficult to determine whether Clouds move in a Direction exactly parallel to the Plane of the Horizon: and it is much more probable that they are in a perpetual Change, *encreafing* or *melting*; rifing or falling, according to the *Preffure* and fpecific Gravity of the *Medium* in which they float; its Tendency to Moifture or Drinefs, Cold or Heat; alfo the different Combinations and Decompofitions, with Refpect to which, the Atmofphere is in perpetual Variation.

The Motion of Trees, if carefully attended to, feldom fhew Effects of a regular horizontal Current.

And fince the more *powerful* the Wind; the more evident and accurate may be the Obfervation; it will be found, that the *firft* general Effect is an oblique Depreffion, fucceeded by a Recovery or inftant Exaltation: then a momentary Paufe, or actual Retreat of the Wind; and in a few Seconds, a Return of the depreffing Torrent.

But the ftrongeft, and, at the fame Time, an irrefragable Proof, is by *Appeal* to Men of *Science* in the Navy, or to fkilful Pilots, who are converfant with Winds and Waves; who have weathered Storms off Cape Hatteras in Latitude 36; (where probably the Wind is perpetual;) or have made an Eaft-India Voyage:—whether, if a Gale blew in an horizontal Direction ONLY; the Ocean coud produce fuch an Inequality of Surface:

Surface: or whether when the Sea runs MOUN-TAINS *high*; the tremendous Surges must not arise from the *violent* Action of Winds repeated at Intervals, sometimes *descending* perpendicularly; but oftener in forcible elastic Torrents of oblique DEPRESSION, and instant *Resilition?*

CHAPTER XXXXV.

Section 243. INtimations of depressing Columns in moderate Weather, are the *sluggish* Clouds, which often make their *first* Appearance, and remain longest, nay almost continually, *over* and *along* great Rivers, and Chains of Mountains, both during a Calm, or from whatever Point the Wind blows. *A gentle Depression of Air over moist Places in fair Weather.*

And hence the greater Quantity, Violence, and Continuance of Wind and Rain, which then *descend* (a): also of the *greater* Purity of the Air *during* such Descent.

244. As, therefore, it is plain that atmospheric Air DESCENDS *frequently*, both in bad and fine Weather; if a Cause can be assigned so general, as to make it probable, that such DEPRESSION does almost continually take Place:—tho' at present the Effect is only evident to the Senses, by actual Experiment in the Passage of Balloons throu' such Columns;—it will be sufficient to put
Balloonists

(a) The Depression and Reverberation of the Wind near Rivers, and its Descent from Mountains, *a Point to be discussed*, may furnish a Hint and Reason, why Rain falls more in one Place, than in another not far distant: and why in the same Place it falls in different Quantities, at different Heights, irregularly.

Balloonifts on their Guard againſt the Effects of ſuch *Depreſſion.*

245. In order to inveſtigate the Theory of Depreſſion; it may not be unacceptable, particularly to thoſe who have not had Leiſure to peruſe the Experiments on Air, by Dr. Prieſtley, or the Collection on the ſame Subject by Cavallo;—juſt to extract a few ſhort Quotations, on the chemical Affinities of Air and Water.

246. Article 1. " Water, as Rain, imbibes only the pure Air of the upper Regions, leaving the lighter and floguiſticated Air to aſcend." (*a*)

246. 2. Felicè Fontana ſays, " Common Air receives an Encreaſe of Bulk and *Elaſticity* from being ſhaken in Water." (*b*)

246. 3. Air abſorbs Water, and Water abſorbs Air: (*c*) and the Abſorption of Air by Water is promoted by Agitation: it alſo abſorbs twice as much *defloguiſticated* Air, as common Air: (*d*) the whole Bulk of the Air abſorbed being equal to one-twelfth of the Bulk of the Water: yet the Bulk of the Water ſeems but *little* encreaſed: the Air being contained within the Interſtices of the Water.

247. The following is a pretty and an eaſy Experiment, to ſhew how the ABSORPTION OF WATER BY AIR takes Place, under the immediate Inſpection of the Obſerver.

Admitting the Sun's Light into a Room, throu' one Window only; pour a Pint of *boiling* Water into a large Baſon: hold the Baſon, which will not be half full, next the Light, in ſuch a Manner,

---

(*a*) Cavallo's Treatiſe on Air, Page 446.——(*b*) 442.——(*c*) 441.——(*d*) 442.

ner, that the Sun may shine on the Water and Bason; yet the Eyes be shaded by the Top of the Window Frame.

Incline the Side of the Bason towards the Light, so that the Water may rise even with the Top.

The Eye being placed just above the upper Side of the Bason, farthest from the Light; look on the Water.

You may then observe the Surface of the Water next the Light, refract the Sun's Rays, and produce the primary Colours, particularly the RED and GREEN: which tho' *transient, continue* to be *seen* in Succession; as Vapours rise above the Surface of the Water. Their *first* Ascent is plainly discoverable: remaining above its Surface, in the Form of *small Dust*, gently agitated, not *separately* but as a *whole*. Nor do they seem to rise into Steam, till assisted by the Action, and Contact of *dry Air*, which like *dry* Spunges, *licks off* and absorbs the small Dust already accumulated by the Force of the Heat from below, and then becomes visible, under the Appearance of Steam, flying off in distinct hollow Vesicles.

The more *still* the Air of the Room, the more slowly will the Spunges of Air come in Contact with the Body of small Dust.—Besides the small Dust already mentioned; the Heat will detach solid Globules of Water; which will remain floating on the Surface of the Body of Water: till the dry Air descends and transports them with it; the Air at the same Instant dissolving the solid Globules into hollow Vesicles.

But the most extraordinary Phenomenon, and which cannot be mistaken, is, that as soon as a

Spunge

Spunge of Air has dipped into the Surface of Water, and received its Lading; the Vesicles continue to accumulate, till another fresh Spunge descends in a similar Form, which may be traced upon the Surface of the Water, and seen in its Shadow, or rather in Beams of Light at the Bottom of the Bason, at the Instant it has flown off with its Burden: for that Part of the Surface of the Water transmits new Rays of Light, on Removal of the Vapour carried away by the Dip and Play of Air.

248. The Removal of the Vapour, likewise exhibits a curious Appearance on the Surface of the Water: which seems as if divided into irregular Parcels detached from each other; like the reticular Daplings visible on the under Side of Clouds elevated to the highest Stratum of the Atmosphere, and there evaporating or dissolving.

249. So powerful is the Attraction between Air and Water; that, while the Steam is rising above and round the Sides of the Bason; *Waves of fresh Air*, by Intervals, press the exterior Parts of the Steam *inwards*, in order to get at the Surface by descending into the Bason.

This Operation is best discovered, when the Bason is held *even*. And the whole Process may be observed more distinctly, if the Bason is raised and fixed on a Frame, near the Height of the Eye of the Observer, standing upright: who will then be able to trace minutely the exact Form of the Steam, and Insinuation of the Waves of Air into the Center of each Curl, or rising Curvature: an Appearance, similar to which, may be seen in *Water* flowing from a small Orifice in a close Vessel;

Veffel; the frefh Air forcibly entering in an oppofite Direction; forming a vifible Cavity and Curvature in the Center of the Stream. See Halley's Experiments on Evaporation in the open Air, and in a clofe Room, in Lowthorp's Abridgement of the Phil. Tranf. Vol. 2, P. 108.

Having once remarked the foregoing Procefs at Leifure; the fame may be feen over any open Veffel of Water juft warm enough to emit vifible Steam: but the Air fhoud be as *ftill* and *calm* as poffible: the Steam never rifing from all Parts of the Surface at once; but a depreffing Spunge of Air always defcends to the Surface, the Inftant a Lamina of Vapour has been detached.

Such is the regular and invariable Procefs of Evaporation.

The fame Procefs may be diftinctly traced over the Surface of a Piece of Water or River, the Air being perfectly calm, in a gentle Froft, at Sunrife, particularly in Autumn, while the Water retains a Warmth fuperior to that of the Air.

250. Hence it follows that *as much light* (*a*) and *warm* Air as is raifed with the Steam by Evaporation from the Surface of any Water; *fo much heavy* and *cool* Air is INSTANTANEOUSLY, conftantly, and forcibly DEPRESSED upon its Surface, in order to fupply the Vacancy, reftore the Equilibrium, and continue the Evaporation. (*b*)

251. Now,

(*a*) It is *light* in Confequence of its *Warmth*, when compared with the *cooler condenfed Air* above it.

(*b*) In the fame Manner that Curls and Streams of Air *defcended* into the Bafon over the rifing *Steam*, and interrupted the Regularity of *its* Elevation; in the *larger* Towns, during Winter *(the Weather being moderate)* the Preffure of Air on all Sides, from without, produces a conftant Breeze towards

251. Now, besides the mutual Affinity that Water has to almost all Kinds of Air, and to Floguiston; added to its Power of Absorption; and as the SEA, particularly in Summer, also RIVERS and *damp* MEADOWS are generally *cooler* than the Lands and Countries bordering on them; Currents of *damp cool* Air press forwards to supply the Defect or Vacancy caused by Heat, Rarefaction and Elevation of *dry warm* Air, which is necessarily, and almost constantly rising into the Atmosphere, from heated Lands, Plains, and gentle Eminences *long shone* on by the Sun.

252. Consequently the pure, cool, defloguisticated Atmosphere, is almost continually descending from above; sometimes imperceptibly, often forcibly, wards the Center of the Town: as may be discovered, not only by the Smoke in its Deviation from the Perpendicular, as it issues from the Chimneys; but by all who are inclined to make the Trial; for, on leaving the Town, they will *meet* the Breeze.

In calm Weather, during Summer, the contrary Event happens: but more particularly in *hot* Climates. For the Country being hotter than the Town; a *Depression* of the Atmosphere takes Place, and scatters the Smoke on all Sides round the Town.

The Cities in Italy, and other hot Climates, on Account of the Buildings, and *desirable* Narrowness of the Streets, form *one* contiguous *Shelter, Arbor,* or grand *Parasol*: For which Reason, the Nobility leave the Country, and reside in the Towns during Summer: there finding a Coolness and Refreshment unknown on the *scorching* Plains.

A *Reception* and *Dispersion* of Air takes Place; *as will presently be mentioned.*

The same ocular Proof and Process in the Evaporation of Steam, accounts at once, for a curious Phenomenon constantly observable on all Waters; viz. *a narrow* SMOOTH *irregular Surface of considerable Length, nearly in the Direction of the Wind, yet unaffected by it*: all which is probably nothing more than *rising* Volumes of *elastic invisible* Steam; *resisting* the *two* nearest *descending Waves* of AIR; and preventing them from approaching the *Surface* of Water, over which the Steam is compressed; and *there* producing a *temporary* CALM.

forcibly, on the Surface of the Sea, the Channels of Rivers, Meadows, and all wet Land. Which Depreſſion acts, in Proportion to its Strength, on the Balloon; and always with a ſenſible Effect: for, being in Equilibrio with the Air at all ſtationary Heights; the *leaſt* Depreſſion of the Atmoſphere makes the Balloon deſcend, conſiderably.

253. This Reaſoning is, in many Caſes, applicable to the Air, and conſequently the Weather and Cold of Mountains.

Nor can it otherways be accounted for, why the Snow is perpetual, and the Cold ſo intenſe, on Mountains under the Equinoctial, and between the Tropics: but which admits an eaſy Solution on the above Hypotheſis. (*a*)

CHAPTER

(*a*) Phil. Tranſ. for 1777, Page 470. Thibet in Lat. 31, *cold* with Snow and Froſt.

See Ulloa's Voyage to South-America, Book 6, Chapter 7; where he deſcribes the ſnowy Mountains, under the Equator.

As the Weather, near the Equinoctial, is more regular, its Changes cloſely following thoſe of the Moon; and alſo the Winds and Hurricanes more violent; the Truth of the foregoing Theory will receive the ſtrongeſt Confirmation by tracing the Effects of DEPRESSING TORRENTS OF AIR, in the Iſland of Jamaica, extracted from the Author already mentioned.

" The cool Vapour *ruſhes* from the Mountains towards the hot dry Air, which hovers over the Savannahs or Vallies.

The Rain falls heavieſt in the Mountains. Vol. 3, Page 600.

The *Land-Wind* after Rain, proceeds from that Quarter whence the Rain has fallen *heavieſt*; and ſeems to *ruſh* from above.

In Spain and North-America, the Wind *ruſhes down*. Page 601.

When the *Land* is *moſt* heated, the Sea-Breeze blows almoſt *all* Night. Page 602.

The Barometer ſubſides from 1 Inch to $1\frac{1}{2}$ *at* the full Moon, or juſt *after* it.

Wind blows from the Mountains all round the Iſland; and
ſtill

CHAPTER XXXXVI.

Section 254. THE Subject of DEPRESSING TORRENTS requires an accurate

ſtill a Sea-Breeze over the Mountains: to the Low-Lands, none, 604.

(In Jamaica likewiſe the Wind blows off the Iſland *every way* at once, ſo that no Ship can any where come in by Night, or go out but early in the Morning, before the Sea-Breeze ſets in. See Abr. Phil. Tr. Vol. 3, P. 548.)

Mountain Air ruſhes down in a continual Current to every Part of the Coaſt, the Stream deſcending inceſſantly throu' the Night: while heavy cold Air deſcends to the Mountain Tops, 604.

With a *Weſt* Wind below there is an *Eaſt Scud above,* 605. Mountains CLOUDY, low Lands SUNNY, 606.

In ALL the River-Courſes of *Jamaica, there is a ſenſible Current of Air. Rain never comes without ſome Wind: and the Showers almoſt invariably follow the very Meanders of the larger Rivers,* 608.

Rain always cools: the Thermometer falling, after a Shower, from 6 to 8 Degrees, 610.

(And Iron ruſts leaſt in rainy Weather: [the Air being then DRIEST,] deſcending from the *upper* Regions. Abr. Ph. Tr. V. 3 P. 546.)"

It is ſaid alſo that " in Jamaica the Clouds gather, and *ſhape* according to the Mountains: ſo that *old Seamen* will tell you each *Iſland* towards Evening, by the *Shape* of the Cloud *over it.*"

The Sea-Breeze, being counterpoiſed by *Deſcent* of the *etherial Air,* produces a CALM.

The ſame Author likewiſe ſays, that " the Clouds begin to gather about 2 or 3 o'Clock in the Afternoon *at the Mountains,* and do not *embody* firſt in the Air, and after ſettle there, but *ſettle* firſt and *embody* there: the reſt of the Sky being clear till *Sun-ſet.* So that they do not paſs *near* the Earth in a *Body,* and only *ſtop* where they meet with Parts of the Earth elevated *above the reſt*; but PRECIPITATE *from a very great Height,* and in Particles of an *exceeding rarified Nature; ſo as not to obſcure the Air or Sky at all:* that great Variety of beautiful Colours in the Canopy of Heaven being raiſed to a much greater Diſtance [he means Height] in Jamaica than it is here." Abr. Ph. Tr. V. 3, P. 557.

(Prognoſtics of Weather, at certain Periods of the Moon, are mentioned by Captain Langford. Lowthorp's Abr. Phil. Tranſ. Vol. 2, Page 105.)

curate Inveſtigation: as it will ſerve to point out the proper Time of Day or Night, when an Aironaut ought ſo to calculate his Voyage, as to arrive over the Middle of the Channel, or Arm of the Sea, at ſome particular Hour: in order to wait for a Sea Breeze which may waft him to the other Side.

A Point not difficult to be aſcertained.

Alſo, this Idea of DEPRESSION, if properly conſidered and digeſted; may prove a ſufficient Foundation on which to eſtabliſh a new Theory of the *Weather*, ſo ill determined at preſent, from its *aggregate Weight* or *Elaſticity* only, as indicated by the Barometer.

255. If a Conjecture may be formed on a Subject, material in itſelf, yet of which ſo little is actually known; woud not *the proper Time* of undertaking a Voyage over the Channel be ſuch, that the Aironaut ſhoud find himſelf three Parts of the Way acroſs, by NINE *o'Clock* in the Morning?

256. In *warmer* Climates, where the Seaſons are more regular; the *Land-Breeze* blows to Sea from Midnight till X. in the Morning: at which Time, the *Sea-Breeze* blows to Land; continues till V. or VI. in the Evening; and is ſucceeded by a CALM, which laſts till Midnight.

Whence it follows, that during the Time of the Sea-Breeze, there is a conſtant Tendency towards a GULPH OF AIR, *along the Middle* of the Channel: the Equilibrium of which is as conſtantly ſupplied by a *Depreſſion* of the upper and in general cooler Strata of Air; and therefore a *dangerous* Time for the Paſſage of Balloons.

On

On the contrary, during the Night, and till ten in the Morning, there is an *Accumulation* of Air, *along the Middle of the Channel:* which confequently is a proper Time to enfure a *fafe* Paffage; by the Affiftance of WINGS, or fome PROPULSIVE Machinery.

Of the horizontally calm medioceanal depreffing Current.

257. The Deficiency or Vacuity being fupplied from the etherial Regions; it might be taken for granted, that fuch Ether muft be *confiderably* lighter than the adjacent common Air on an equal Level, and therefore *proportionably* dangerous for the Paffage of Balloons.

But if it be confidered that fuch Air, acting as a WEDGE, or more probably in the Form of an hyperbòlic Solid, (*a*) to fill up the Vacuity, defcends with Rapidity from a *colder* Atmofphere impregnated with aqueous Vapours *invifible from below*; and that both the Air and Vapour have reciprocal Affinities and Attractions, electric and mechanical, with the Body of Water beneath them; and are often rendered ftill cooler by its conftant Agitation and *Evaporation*; alfo, that the Supply being immediate and cotemporary, with the DOUBLE TIDE OF AIR flowing from the *middle* over the *oppofite* Shores;—there poffibly may be little or no Difference between the aggregate or *barometric* Gravity of *fuch* Columns, and thofe which are formed by the Sea-Breeze on either Side of them: therefore the Defcent of Balloons

---

(*a*) The Depreffion of a *Torrent* of Air in the Form of an hyperbolic Solid, *contracting* as it *defcends* to the Earth, in Proportion as its *Denfity* encreafes; may furnifh a Hint towards the Solution of a Difficulty how to account for the Augmentation of veficulous Vapours into large folid Drops, frequent during *Summer-*Showers.

loons is owing, among other Causes, to an almost perpendicular actual Depression of the superincumbent Atmosphere (*a*).

Following up the Idea of a Sea-Breeze, blowing, at a Medium, for 20 Miles over Land; altho' the Stratum of the LOWER CURRENT of Air, or Sea Breeze, may not exceed HALF A MILE IN DEPTH, measuring from the Ground upwards; nearly equal to 26 Inches of the Barometer *above*, the Thermometer also *above* being at 55, i. e. *Temperate:*—yet this Observation may prove of essential Service, while the UPPER CURRENT of Air, i. e. the general Wind blows TOWARDS the Sea, (which will be found to take Place more *frequently* than is, at present, imagined;) or while the Balloon is influenced that Way; as was the Case with Sadler and his Companion when over the Nore: who, on his accidental and sudden Descent, fortunately found Safety in the SEA-BREEZE.

Which Breeze was sought for, and made Use of by the Author, when in the Balloon, near Frodsham, in Cheshire.

For, as the Sea-Breeze is pretty general, Aironauts shoud not be too apprehensive: as they have it in their Power, by proper Management, to drop into the Breeze—for EITHER SHORE: if they are provided with a Machinery to waft themselves across the intermediate *depressing* or *accumulating* MEDIOCEANAL COLUMN OF AIR:
which

(*a*) Monf. Sauffure's valuable " Essais sur L'Hygrometrie," throw new Light on the Doctrine of Rarefaction and Condensation not unfavourable to the Hypothesis here advanced. Page 260.

which Space, between the two Shores, is, as before hinted, frequently BECALMED.

258. Further: as the above Theory of a *medioceanal* Depreſſion ſeems to receive additional Confirmation from *each* Balloon Experiment; Lunardi *deſcending* on the 5th of October laſt, when near the Middle of the Bay of Edinburgh or Frith of Forth;—it may be found *prudent*, to keep the Balloon continually riſing, till the Aironaut is *one-third* of the Paſſage *over*.

258. 2. For if the general Wind in the upper Current be not ſtrong; the Aironaut may expect to be *becalmed*, with Reſpect to the horizontal Direction of the Current, the Inſtant he finds, by the Riſe of the Barometer, that the Balloon *deſcends*; i. e. when it is acted upon by the depreſſing Column: in which Caſe, the *higher* he has ſoared, the *ſafer*: as he will have more Room and greater *Latitude* for Exertion by Means of the Machinery: which Machinery will be greatly *aided* by the Force of the deſcending Column or Gravity; and will act on a ſimilar Principle with the Ferry-Boats over the River Po in Italy; which are a Sort of horizontal Pendulum. For the Aironauts will continue to *deſcend*, at the ſame Time that their *Wings* furniſh the Means of a progreſſive Motion.

Therefore, before the Time that the Balloon has reached the Surface of the Water; they will have croſſed the depreſſing Column; and find themſelves wafted *gently* by the *new* Sea-Breeze ſetting in towards the oppoſite Shore.

259. If the Aironaut *riſes up* to Sea with a Wind blowing from the Land on each of the oppoſite Sides

Sides of the Channel, and arrives above the Middle of the Channel, while the same Wind remains; it is probable that the Balloon will continue to rise higher as he proceeds towards the Middle, *where* the MEDIOCEANAL ACCUMULATION has for some Hours taken Place; and therefore he need not be under any Apprehension of falling: but, as before, it being probable he will also be *becalmed*; the Necessity of propulsive Machinery is equally urgent, in order to pass the Center of the *Accumulation*: after which, the Balloon will ride Home to the opposite Shore in the new Sea-Breeze, by *that* Time, just beginning to set in.

260. With the Assistance of propulsive Machinery, it is imagined the Aironaut may be enabled in a few Minutes to force throu' the calm medioceanal Accumulation, or Depression: after which, he will have little Occasion to make Use of it.

261. SUNRISE is, probably, the SAFEST Time of all, to ascend towards the Sea, with an *Air-tight* Balloon: arriving with the Assistance of the Wings, throu' the *calm* medioceanal Accumulation: and there waiting till the new *Sea-Breeze* sets in to the *opposite* Shore.

CHAPTER XXXXVII.

Difficulties, proposed by Monf. Sauffure stated; and their Solution attempted.

Section 259. IT may be observed here, that the two Difficulties proposed by Sauffure, are, in a great Meafure, removed; in admitting the Doctrine of mediocèanal *Depreffion*, and confequent alternate *Accumulation*.

In a diftinct Chapter, treating of the Variation of the Barometer, which he allows has Need of farther Explanation; he afks (Page 308) what Reafons can be affigned, why the *Eaft* Winds, which are *cold and dry*, make the Barometer *defcend*, in England and Holland: yet, the *Weft* Winds, which are *moift and temperate*, make it *rife*?

The Eaft Winds *here* blow chiefly in Spring.

Now it is univerfally agreed, that the Sea, is fooner heated by the Sun than the Land: and on Account of the marine Acid exhaled, *(a)* is alfo lefs cold, *(b)* during that Seafon, in the fame Latitude.

In

(a) Ice, when expofed to marine acid Air, is diffolved by it, as faft as if it touched a red hot Iron. See Cavallo's Treatife on Air, Page 727. Alfo Prieftley's Experiments and Obfervations, Vol. 1, Page 148.

(b) " The WATER remains TRANSPARENT or colourlefs, tho' faturated with marine acid Air, and by a very gentle Degree of Heat, the Gafs may be again expelled from it, as it is expelled from Spirit of Salt."

This Obfervation is applicable to the Tranfparency of Vapours, in the Air, tho' mixed with the marine Acid exhaled from the Sea: for when the acid or Sea Air is mixed with Alkaline or Land Air, they inftantly *combine*; lofe their Elafticity, and form a *white* vifible Subftance or *Cloud*. Cavallo, Page 728. Prieftley's Exp. and Obf. Vol. 2, Page 293.

In Spring, therefore, the great Atlantic or Weftern Ocean, being *lefs* cold than England, Holland, and Eaftwards; the Air pendent over the moft extenfive Tract of *dry and cool Land* in the World, rufhes Weftwards to fupply the Equilibrium of *warm light* Air rifing upwards, and caufing a temporary medioceanal Accumulation: which (altho' the fpecific Gravity of the cold Air is greater) muft produce an actual Deficiency in the aggregate Weight of the Atmofphere over England and Holland: confequently the Barometer falls.

Again: the Weft Winds which blow at other Seafons; if, in Winter; are not frequent, except about Noon after frofty Nights which have equalized the Air for the Tranfmiffion of vigorous Sunfhine: and fhoud be looked upon as (what they are really obferved to be) *low* partial Sea-Breezes, or EDDY *Currents*, infinuating themfelves near the Surface, and fetting Eaftwards frequently againft the upper and more general Winds; and therefore produce a temporary Accumulation.

If, in Summer; the Supply of cool Air to the heated Land, being made not only from the *Northern Ocean*, and lofty *Mediterranean Mountains*; but alfo from the *Atlantic Breezes*; the latter, tho' *moift and temperate*, muft alfo tend towards an Accumulation of the Atmofphere over England and Holland: and therefore the Barometer rifes.

CHAPTER

CHAPTER XXXXVIII.

Facts and Observations tending to confirm the Doctrine of Accumulation and Depression.

Section 260. BEFORE the Subject of medi-oceànal Accumulation and Depression of Air, is wholly quitted; it may be well to mention and compare a few Facts and Observations, which will elucidate the Doctrine; and in their Turn, receive Light from it.

261. If, in the Middle of a *hot sunny* Day, Vapours lighter than the Air, were to rise from the Ocean, (which they will continue to do, in hollow Vesicles or Bladders, till the Expansion breaks the Bubble, at which Time the Water woud fall to the Earth, if not drank up by the Attraction of *dry* Spunges of Air;) there woud be a constant Wind blowing from *Land to Sea*, to fill up the Chasm: but at such Time, the Land is more heated than the Sea: therefore hot Air and Vapour arise from both; and the Breeze, on the contrary, blows from *Sea to Land*; consequently if the Vacuities were not *continually* supplied from the etherial Regions, and from the Ocean, all Animals woud actually die, for Want of Air, as in a *hot close* Room.

Such Supply is therefore constantly made, by Depression of the Atmosphere, and Absorption of the Water.

262. What happens on a great Scale, above the Ocean, as *before* hinted; probably, happens on a smaller, over Channels or Arms of the Sea: and on a still smaller; over and along Rivers, Brooks, wet Meadows, and damp Grounds.

263. In

263. In the variable Latitudes on the Atlantic Ocean; *cool fresh* Air is supplied from above, by descending Vortices of Wind and Showers: i. e. *Storms* of COLLECTION. (a)

264. It may be remarked, in Confirmation of the above Doctrine, that triangular or Latteen Sails are used, and more useful, in a Mediterranean Sea, surrounded by high Lands, from which the Wind suddenly descends in Squalls; than in the open Atlantic, where the Wind is more equal.

264. 2. Perhaps there cannot be a better Account of the depressing Torrent of Air, than that which Bacon has given, in describing the Motion of Wind on the Sails of Ships, in a *Squall*.

"All Wind acting on the Sails of a Vessel, tends to depress or sink it. Wherefore *in strong Gales*, they first haul down the Yards, and take in the Topsails: afterwards all the Sails: cut away the Masts: throw the Lading overboard, the Guns, &c. to lighten the Vessel, and keep her above Water." (b)

CHAPTER XXXXIX.

Section 265. WITH Respect to Mountains: on reading what Travellers have written, particularly Ullòa; (c) they seem to answer the Intention of supplying cool Air to the surrounding Plains, or Continents; by Depression

Torrents of Air on Etna, and Teneriffe.

(a) On the Descent of Air in *Thunder-Gusts*, see "Chalmer's Account of the Weather in South-Carolina, Vol. 1, Page 1, to 39."
(b) "Historia Ventorum, Pag. 54, Art. 34."
(c) Book V. Chapter 2d.

pression and Condensation: and also, if on Islands; to the Sea itself.

266. Brydone, in his Tour throu' Sicily and Malta, in 1773; (a) giving an Account of his Ascent to the Top of Etna, says, that at the Foot of the Crater, the Snow was frozen hard and solid: (b) and that the Crater was so hot; it was impossible to descend into it.

Further: " that the Smoke rolled down from the Sides, like a Torrent: till of equal Gravity with the Air, when it shot off horizontally; forming a long Track, according to the Direction of the *Wind:* which there rose to a VIOLENT Degree: so that it was with Difficulty he coud settle the Barometer for an Observation."

He also adds " that *Clouds* began to *gather* round the *Mountain*; but were *dispelled* by the Wind."

Now from the foregoing Theory is it not probable to suppose, that a *Torrent of Air rushed* continually down from the etherial Regions, not only to supply the Fire of the Crater; but also the Vacuity caused by the perpetual Elevation of Vapours and heated Air from below: the Torrent likewise *depressing* into the Track with itself, the Volumes of Smoke which were seen to roll directly down the Sides of the Mountain: that this descending Torrent of Air, in its Progress, dispelled the Clouds forming round the Sides of the Mountain, by the Ascent of warm Vapours condensing, as they rose, on their Approach to the cold Mountain: the Smoke shooting *horizontally*,

from

(a) Vol. 1. Page 184.
(b) Page 195.

from that Height *only*, at which an *horizontal Current of Air* began to take Place? For it can hardly be imagined that the Air at the Top of Etna, found to be "*electrical*," and which muſt have been replete with a Mixture of Floguiſton, inflammable Air, Gaſſes, and other aërial Fluids highly rarefied, heated, DRY, (and conſequently lighter,) *at the Inſtant* of riſing out of the glowing Cauldron, became ſo condenſed as to fall like Water, without partaking of the Motion of a *violent* Wind, ſuppoſed to blow in an horizontal Direction.

267. Glas, in his Account of Teneriffe, (*a*) reports, that the Clouds are generally half as high as the Peak, above the Sea (*b*), i. e. according to him, near the Height of a Mile and Half: "*below* which Clouds, the *North Eaſterly Winds* GENERALLY prevail: and, at the ſame Time, *above them*, we find a *freſh Weſterly* GALE: which I believe to be the Caſe *in every Part of the World when the* TRADE WIND *blows.*"

In Page 253, he ſays, that in aſcending above the Level of the Clouds, he found the Air ſharp, cold and piercing: and the Wind blew ſtrong from South Weſt, and Weſt South Weſt: ſo that the Wind blew towards the Mountain from three different Points at leaſt, viz. the Trade Wind,

from

(*a*) Hiſtory of the Canary Iſles, Page 252.
(*b*) As the ſuperior Clouds, during the Balloon Excurſion, did not much exceed the Height of 1000 Yards; ſuppoſing then the Clouds at an equal Height above the Sea, near Teneriffe; one ought to conclude, either, that the Peak was not ſo high as Glas repreſents it; or, that the Level of the Clouds was leſs than half the Height of the Mountain.

from North East below the Clouds; just above them, from South West: and still higher, a fresh Gale, from West.

"The Air on the Top of the Pike was thin, cold, piercing; and of a dry parching Nature, like the South Easterly Winds which I have felt in the great Desert of Africa, or the Levanters in the Mediterranean: or even not unlike those dry easterly Winds which are frequent in the Northern Parts of Europe, in clear Weather, in the Months of March or April," Page 257.

This dry Wind answers to the Eknèfiai (before mentioned) i. e. *Wind descending* FROM THE CLOUDS.

Glas further observes (Page 250) that the Clouds, in fine Weather, descend gradually towards Evening, and rest on the Woods till Morning: when they re-ascend, and remain suspended above them, till the succeeding Evening.

Here then a nocturnal Depression of the Atmosphere is obvious. But this Appearance will not prove that the Air does not descend below the Level of the Clouds: for, tho' the Clouds descend with the Air; Vapour-Air, of which they are composed, becomes *transparent* both by Dissolution, in a warmer Stratum, and Proximity to the Earth, as before mentioned.

Conclusion drawn from the above, applicable to Balloons.

268. From the Variety of Winds experienced at different Heights, not only on *Teneriffe*, but in different Places; it is plain, that if Balloons can be made durable and Air-tight; they may be wafted between the Tropics by an East or West

West Current at Pleasure: and also throu'out the Globe; the Occasion being made, in some Respect, subservient to the Time (*a*).

CHAPTER L.

CORROBORATING PROOFS OF A DEPRESSION.

Sect. 268. Art. 1. THE Author is well informed, that, during an Engagement at Sea;—in *ten* Minutes after the Action has commenced;—tho' it blew a *Gale* before; (that is, tho' it blew *violently*;) the Agitation of the Air, arising from the Explosion of the *great Guns*, and small Arms, woud counteract the Wind, and produce a dead Calm.

268. 2. Quere: does not the *new elastic* Air, produced from the Nitre, (*b*) give an instantaneous Compression and Dilatation to the *incumbent* atmospheric Air, round the Place of Action, while the *lighter floguisticated Air* passes throu' it, raising, and affecting to its highest Limit, the *whole* Atmosphere. And does not the Effect of a sudden Calm, suppose the Wind to *descend from above* with a Kind of *saltatory* Motion, instantly counteracted by the *new elastic* Air ?—For if the Wind be supposed to blow sideways or horizontally,

---

(*a*) See " Royal Astronomer, by R. Heath, Page 321, on *Trade Winds and Monsoons*."

(*b*) One Pound of Nitre only, producing by mere Heat, 6 cubic Feet of Air. " Cavallo, Page 332, and 811, Experiments on Gun-Powder."

zontally, *to any confiderable Height above* the Water, woud not the frefh *lateral* Air glide away, and prevent the Continuance of the Calm?

269. When a Squall happens, or only Rain falls; Air will *rufh* from all Sides, and from *above*, to fupply the Vacancy of the fallen Cloud and Vapour.

The Air immediately *above* muft fall: the lateral Air gravitating towards other Places. Hence *Cold*, and a bright Sky after Rain.

270. The Theory of Accumulation may account for the frequent *warm* Rains in Winter, and during the Night.

For the preceding diurnal Accumulation over the Sea, may *circulate* during the Night, at a great Altitude, to reftore the Equilibrium and Lofs of *cold* Land Air fent by a low or Ground-Wind to Sea, during the Day-Time: particularly, as *the Accumulation* over the Sea, during Winter, is almoft *continual*.

271. The *Wind* would more frequently be perceived to *defcend* and *rebound upwards*, (Trials of which might be made by holding an Umbrella, extended at right Angles with its Axis, upright in the Hand;) if the fame Opportunity offered, of oppofing as great a Surface to it in a perpendicular, as is every Day done, in an horizontal Direction: for in walking, the whole Height of the Body, and half its Surface, is oppofed horizontally to the Wind: but the Head only, which is covered, is oppofed to the perpendicular Preffure.

272. As every Circumftance in the Order of Nature is fo admirably contrived that each apparent Inconvenience rectifies itfelf; in *heavy*
Winds

Winds continuing to blow from a COLD Point; the Conſtruction of the Atmoſphere is ſuch, that the *warm light* Air from the oppoſite Points will neceſſarily riſe up and flow over the cold Stratum, and by their Tendency to an Equilibrium, will produce an Air *leſs cold*, before the *ſame* Wind is exhauſted.

273. On the one Hand; it is probable, that, as cold Winds are heavy; the Eknèfiai Winds are covered with frequent Waves of the Apogay, or light warm Air rolling over them, frequently from the oppoſite Points.

274. On the other Hand, as the *Apogay* Winds are naturally light and warm, it is *improbable* that they ſhoud be *frequently* covered with Waves of *cold heavy Air*, rolling over them from Eknèfiai Points.

It may therefore be reaſonably concluded, that the Eknèfiai Winds, when approaching or oppoſed to the Apogay, ſhoud be conſidered as *Ground Winds*, (i. e. Winds blowing next the Surface of the Earth, tho' they be ſuppoſed at the ſame Time to deſcend) which receive the Apogay above them: and that the Apogay being warm light and MOIST, (which laſt will have the ſame Effect, as if they were more elaſtic;) (*a*) being alſo more turbulent, and endued with greater Velocity, preſs back the Eknèfiai from the Surface of the Earth, and upwards; and at the ſame Time flow above them.

By

(*a*) "See Recherches ſur les Modifications de l'Atmoſphere. No. 715." Ph. Tranſ. Part 2, for 1777. Col. Roy's Experiments, Sect. 2d, Page 689, 744. 753, 764.

By which means the Eknèfiai partake of their Qualities;—become lefs *cold*, lefs *heavy*, and lefs *dry* (*a*).

CHAPTER

(*a*) The different Phenomena of the *Aurora Borealis* may be owing to the Afcent and Motion of the Apogay, in the *middle* Region, over the Stratum of Eknefiai or *Ground-*Winds.

The Effects of *Tides in the Air yet to be* mentioned, muft not, however, be wholly excluded.

The Aurora Borealis is feen in *Spring, Autumn,* and *Winter :* fometimes *culminating,* fometimes moving in *Streams* and *Waves* in the *fuperior* Regions of the Atmofphere: when culminating; as if rifing out of Clouds in the North.

This Appearance may be owing to warm moift Air perpetually generating between the Tropics, and rolling over the cold *dry* Stratum of Eknèfiai Winds, which cut off its Communication with the Earth ; till accumulating over the Poles, it enlightens the Atmofphere, converting a fix *Month*'s *Night* into Day; and returns to the Surface filently: or in Lightning, whenever it is communicated to the Earth, throu' *Vapour defcending* hy its own fpecific Gravity; or along with *depreffing* Torrents of Air, known to be accompanied by frequent FLASHES.

When the Vapour is *condenfed* in its Defcent, by paffing throu' a Stratum of the Eknèfiai Winds; it becomes *overcharged* with the electric Matter, *furrounding* and *adhering* to it; and depofits the Overplus in Lightning, on its Approach to *other* Clouds, or to the *Earth.*

It is vifible in the Form of a Vapour, when the Vapour to which it adheres, becomes overcharged with electric Matter, by Defcent into a *cool* Eknèfiai Stratum below : there forming a luminous and tranfparent Atmofphere: the Particles of Light and Vapour being repelled to great Diftances from each other at fo *rare* a Height.

It culminates above the Vapour, becaufe lefs heavy than the circumambient Air ; and may be fubject to the Attraction of other Planets.

The Aurora Borealis is alfo feen to iffue in Streams and Waves of Light, with inexpreffible Velocity, on its Return to the South, in a lower Stratum, as it *paffes throu*' Interftices, between the Veficles of warm Vapour, raifed and difperfed by the turbulent Apogay Winds, in the middle Region.

During Summer, the middle Region becomes blended with the lower, throu' Defect of Cold ; and the electric Matter is fuppofed to be communicated to the Earth, filently, and continually ; but by Lightning, when a lower and colder Atmofphere

CHAPTER LI.

Section 275. IF then this Reasoning be allowed; aërial Travellers will not be subject, when, at a considerable Height, even in Winter, to great Degrees of Cold, supposing that the Air does not actually freeze the Waters below; and the Apogay or Southerly Winds have continued for a few Days.

On the Contrary; Aironauts may expect Cold, encreasing with their Ascent, even in Summer, tho' *warm* below; supposing the Eknèfiai or Northerly Winds to have continued but for a Day before the Ascent: they may possibly, indeed by soaring higher, rise into the regular Stratum of the warm Apogay floating above them.

276. From what has been said, there seems a Degree of Probability, that the Air for a Number of Miles, *above warm cultivated Plains* shoud differ materially in its Temperature, from Air above Mountains, or *even on a Level* with their Summits.

That the former Air, in moderate Weather, shoud continue *warm and rarefied*: while the latter is *cool and condensed*.

For the same Reason the Air over the Sea, on the Hours of Accumulation; i.e. during the Night, in Summer, and frequently in Winter, shoud

---

mosphere condenses and overcharges the Vapour, and cuts off the Communication.

It cannot be seen but in escaping from Vesicle to Vesicle: nor, during Summer, after Sunset, on Account of the Twilight.

shoud be found *warm* and *rarefied:* especially during a Continuance of the Apogay Winds.

277. It is likewise probable that the Atmosphere will be found RESPIRABLE at much greater Heights, than is at present imagined: during the Continuance of the Eknèfiai Winds; and also, on Account of the *defloguisticated* Air, (*a*) which is *drier* and *less elastic* in Proportion to its Rarity. (*b*)

278. The Height of 10 Miles seems not too great to limit human Respiration, shoud any Attempt be made, to soar with a Balloon in a mild Atmosphere; and particularly between the Tropics. (*c*).

Balloon:

(*a*) Air is not unfit for Respiration, by having lost its *vital* Principle, but because it has imbibed *Floguiston,* which cannot easily be separated from it, but by Agitation in Water. Cavallo. on Air, Pages 479, 670.

(*b*) For if Moisture be one Cause, which keeps the Particles of Air at greater Distances from each other; this Cause decreases at *great* Altitudes.

If also the *Elasticity* decreases in Proportion, not only to the Height, but the Driness; its Particles must, on both Accounts, approach each other, at great Altitudes: tho', from the Altitude only; they woud separate according to the Rule, viz. that the Rarity of the Air is proportionable to the Relaxation of the Force compressing it.

So that at the Height of 8 or 10 Miles, a Quantity of Air taken from the Surface of the Earth, woud occupy 6 Times its former Space: supposing the Air both below and above to be of the *same Kind,* as well as of the *same mean* Temperature of 55, on the Thermometer. See " Martin's Philosophical Grammar, Page 178."

(*c*) Chalmer describing a Whirlwind, which is a *Storm* of COLLECTION and *Ascent* of HOT Air, &c. by Rarefaction, says, " as the Wind ceased, presently after the Whirlwind passed, the BRANCHES and Leaves of various Sorts of Trees, which had been carried into the Air, continued to FALL for HALF AN HOUR; and, in their Descent, appeared like Flocks of Birds of different Sizes."

This Circumstance proves that Columns of HOT Air must have been raised in a Body, in Succession, to so considerable a Height, that *Branches* of Trees carried up by them, took *half an Hour* in falling.

But an Objection woud be found in the Size of a Balloon fufficiently capacious to contain nearly 6 Times the Bulk to which the Gafs woud neceffarily expand itfelf, at the Height of 10 Miles.

279. It feems moft likely that the primary Caufe that will affect the Afcent of Balloons is the Difficulty of encreafing the Dimenfion of the Balloon: the Second, is from the exceffive Cold; if the Wind blows from any Points of the North. *First Caufe of Limitation, in the Afcent of Balloons. Second Caufe of Limitation in the Afcent of Balloons.*

Suppofing the Conftruction of the Atmofphere to be as reprefented by different Authors, (which, by the Way, is fcarcely credible) ten Miles will perhaps be the utmoft attainable Height.

280. There is a Circumftance relative to the Motion of the Air, which has not been fufficiently attended to: and bears fome Analogy with that of a *Thorough Air*.

This Circumftance may not improperly be called the *Reception* and *Difperfion of Air*.

In cold Climates, it is an Object of Dread: in warm ones, a moft defirable Piece of Luxury.

A gentle Undulation of the Air is perceived in Peru, and other hot Climates, by Perfons fitting in *Arbours* fheltered from the Sun.

The furrounding Air is inftantly *contracted* by *Condenfation*, during the Abfence of the Sun's Rays, and therefore occupies a *lefs* Space: *frefh Air* is *received*, and as inftantly *difperfed* by Expanfion towards thofe Parts, which are the warmeft, i. e. where there is leaft Refiftance: fo that a gentle

Breeze

Breeze is conſtantly kept up, *probably* by a Depreſſion from *above* (a).

281. Analagous to this, are thoſe Winds which generally *riſe early* and die away at *Sunſet:* the nocturnal Condenſation of the Air being ſufficient for the RECEPTION: as Air ſuffers ſome Compreſſion without Tumult.

To demonſtrate the Changes owing alſo to remote and inviſible Cauſes leaſt ſuſpected; Boyle ſomewhere ſpeaks of an Inſtrument he made, which was ſo nicely contrived, that he coud tell, while ſitting in his own Apartment, whenever any detached Cloud paſſed beneath the Sun's Diſk. The Principle on which it acted ſeems to have been that of a Reception and Diſperſion of Air that took Place within *the* SHADOW proceeding from the Cloud.

282. An oblique Argument ſupporting the Doctrine of Depreſſion, aſſerted to take Place, in fair Weather, is that *Wind* drys up the Moiſture from the Ground more than the *Sun:* and that March which is the *windieſt*, is alſo the *moſt drying*, tho' *not* the *hotteſt* Month.

Bacon, in his Enquiry into Motions and Undulations of the Air, uſes a Metaphor, which tho' ſomewhat facetious, is ſtrictly philoſophical. (b) " *For when* WINDS *lead* THE DANCE, *it woud be agreeable to know the* FIGURE." (c)

And

(a) It may be from this Principle, that in the Eaſt, Liquids are kept *cool* by being hung in the Shade, in the *open* Air, ſuſpended in *wet Cloths:* there being a continual Breeze and Succeſſion of COOL DRY *Spunges* (as it were) of Air, in Contact with the *wetted* Cloths, whoſe Moiſture will thus be more quickly evaporated.

(b) Hiſtoria Ventorum, Pag. 48, Art. 33.

(c) " Cum enim (Venti) Choreas ducant, Ordinem Saltationis noſſe jucundum fuerit. Art. 18."

And it is probable, that they really prefs the Earth with a faltatory progreffive undulating Motion, *defcending* in elaftic Steps of fudden Compreffion; and *rifing* with quick alternate ones, of Dilatation and Expanfion.

Dicker's Balloon gave Proof of this.

283. Laftly: the CHILL *of Air* which always takes Place over WATER, and *moift* Grounds, even in the FINEST WEATHER, ftrongly favours the *Reception* and *Difperfion* of *it*, to the furrounding and more heated Lands: (which can only be fupplied, as before mentioned, by Torrents of frefh Air *gradually defcending* from the etherial or middle Region of the Atmofphere;) and feems to produce the fame Effect, viz. a conftant Breeze, with that of the Arbor, Shade, or Shelter from the *Sun:* alfo with that of the *Shadow* from the Cloud paffing under his Difk, which affected a complete Thermometer and Hygrometer.

284. On a Change of Weather from Froft to Thaw, the Colour of the *upper Air* FIRST alters from a *clear and deep*, to a *dull and faint* Blue, or to a muddy Haze, not diftinguifhable into Clouds, but vifible above them; a vivid Brightnefs ftill remaining, for many Hours, to about 500 Yards above the Surface of the Earth.

Or, foft *warm* Showers fall gently, without Wind, or any apparent Change in its Direction.

All which feem to favour the Accumulation and Defcent of *warm Air*, by Waves of the Apogay rolling over the Eknèfiai Winds.

Ff   CHAPTER

CHAPTER LII.

Proper Days in the Month for the Ascent of Balloons.

Section 285. AS the *safest Hour* of the Day has been already pointed out, for the Ascent of those Aironauts, who propose to cross a Channel, or Arm of the Sea, in a Balloon *Air-tight* or nearly so: it may not be useless to throw out a few Hints on the properest Days in *each Month*, for the Ascent of Balloons.

286. It will perhaps be found true, that the more frequent Winds are generated near the Surface of the Earth: but that *Storms* are generated from above. Cold, Heat, Drought, and Moisture produce the more frequent and diurnal Winds: but the Conjunctions and Operations of the Moon and Planets contribute to the Production of Storms and other Inequalities of the Atmosphere: more especially the *Moon*: at the New and Full. These Attractions first affect the *superior Parts* of the Atmosphere. (*a*)

287. "We are sure in the calmest Weather, to have some Breeze at Noon, and at full Tide." Therefore, both are improper Times for Balloons to be at Sea: the Time of low Water and Midnight woud be best in those, if equal in other Respects.

Changes of Weather as to Wind or Calm happen about the New and Full Moon. (*b*)

288 Varieties

(*a*) On the Action of the Sun and Moon over Animal Bodies, by Dr. Mead, Miscell. Cur. Vol. 1. P. 372, 373.

(*b*) For these Observations see Gassendus's Natural Philosophy. De Chales's Navigator. And Astro-Meteoro-Logica, per J. Goad.

288. Varieties of Tide produced by the united or divided Forces of the Sun and Moon, occafion fimilar Changes in the Atmofphere nearly at the fame Time.

For Inftance, at the Time of the New Moon or Conjunction, i. e. when the Earth, Moon, and Sun, are *nearly* in a Line; the Moon being between them: alfo at the Time of the Full Moon; i. e. when the Moon, Earth, and Sun are *nearly* in a Line; and the Earth between them, which is called the Oppofition. (*a*)

In the firft Cafe, the Moon and Sun attract the Atmofphere of the Earth conjointly, or with united Force: in the fecond Cafe; the Earth being between them, they act in Oppofition to each other, ftill nearly in the fame Line.

At thefe Times, the SPRING *Tides* are at the *higheft* i. e. once every Fortnight; and in the two interval Weeks are the NEAP or *loweft* Tides: for a like Reafon.

Becaufe, in the latter Cafe, a Line fuppofed to be drawn from the Moon to the Earth, and another from the Earth to the Sun, woud form nearly a right Angle: or in other Words; becaufe the Moon and Sun woud attract the Earth at right Angles to each other, or in a lateral Direction :—the Moon woud draw one Way and the Sun another :—their Forces woud be divided.

Now it is a Fact, that the Ocean is raifed confiderably twice every twenty-five Hours, by the Attraction of the Moon, when fhe comes to

---

(*c*) See Maclaurin's Newton, Page 376.

the Meridian. So that the Surface of the Sea, instead of putting on the Form of a Sphere, or Globe, will be changed into an *oval* Figure, whose longest Diameter being produced, woud pass throu' the Moon.

In like Manner a similar Elevation must take Place, as often as the Sun is in the Meridian; either above or below the Horizon.

Moreover, this Elevation is *greatest* on the New and Full Moon, because the Moon and Sun do then conspire in their Attractions: and *least* in the Quarters: as they will then draw different Ways; the *Difference* of their Actions only producing an Effect.

Lastly, the Intumescence will be of a *middle* Degree, at the Times between the Quarters, and New and Full Moon.

289. As in the Ocean, so in the Air above it; a Tide of Air must roll along the Atmosphere, throu' the whole Extent of it; and rise upwards twice in about 24 Hours.

And since the Height of the Atmosphere is computed by Halley at 45 Miles, and the Depth of the Ocean at an Average, but half a Mile; the Air will more easily and quickly obey the Attraction of the Moon and Sun, than the Tide of the Ocean: and, as it revolves in a Sphere which is about 100 Times larger than that of the Ocean, the Agitation and the Velocity of its Tide, will be something greater, in Proportion to its Elasticity, and inferior Density to the Water of the Ocean. *(a)*

290. The

(a) Air at a Medium is 800 Times rarer than Water: so that if 800 Times the Quantity of Air *naturally* contained

290. The *Weight* of the Air muſt now be conſidered.

The Weight of the Atmoſphere in England does not exceed $31\frac{1}{2}$ Inches of Mercury in the Barometer: nor does the leaſt Weight fall ſhort of $28\frac{1}{2}$: the greateſt Difference in the Weights may be taken at 2 Inches: dividing 30 (nearly equal to the whole Weight) by 2, the Anſwer is 15. So that the under Parts of the Atmoſphere being preſſed upon by about a fifteenth Part leſs Weight at one Time, than at another; the *ſpecific Gravity* of the Air will ſometimes be a fifteenth Part lighter.

But the Height of the Atmoſphere being eſtimated at 45 Miles, which is equipoiſed by about 30 Inches; when equipoiſed by a fifteenth Part leſs Weight; (that is, dividing 45 Miles by 15; which amounts to the ſame as if a fifteenth Part of the whole Height was taken away; the Anſwer is 3 Miles;) ſhews that the Atmoſphere is 3 Miles higher at one Time than at another, over certain Places; indicated by the Barometer at thoſe Places.

Such an Accumulation of Air, ariſing only from Preſſure or ſpecific Gravity in one Part of the Atmoſphere, and not in another; by its Tendency to an Equilibrium; and when to this Tendency is added its *elaſtic* Force;—muſt be productive of WINDS, *deſcending Torrents*, Inundations of Air, or Storms, near the Surface of the Earth: and nearly ſuch a Difference in the Barometer

---

tained in a Veſſel whoſe Dimenſions are thoſe of a cubic Foot, were preſſed into it by a Syringe or *Condenſer*; the Air woud differ nothing from Water in Denſity.

Barometer has been known to happen in a few Hours.

Such Accumulation, however, is not properly the *Tide of Air*.

291. At the New and Full Moon, the united Attractions of the Moon and Sun raise the Spring Tides in the Ocean to the average Height of 10 Feet and a half. *(a)*

And in the Moon's Quarters, the Moon drawing one Way, while the Sun draws another, viz. at a right Angle, made by Lines from the Sun and Moon to the Earth's Center; the average Height of the Neap Tides in the Ocean will be 6 Feet 7 Inches.

The same Attraction which raises Water 10 Feet and a half, will raise Air, whose Density is 800 Times less, to almost one third of that to which the whole Pressure of the Atmosphere can raise Fluids: *(b)* Now it has been before seen, that the Pressure of the Atmosphere raised the Air 45 Miles: so that the Air is raised by the united Actions of the Moon and Sun, at the New and Full Moon, to one-third Part of 45; i. e. to 15 Miles. And for the same Reason, the Air is raised at the Moon's Quarters to 10 Miles: *(c)* the Difference between which is 5 Miles.

There is consequently a real *Tide of Air* five Miles higher at each New and Full Moon, than at her Quarters: which Tide rolls with incredible

---

(a) See Wilson on Climate, Chap. 15. Pages 46, 54.——
(b) 55.
(c) By reducing 10 Feet 6 Inches, and 6 Feet 7 Inches, into Inches, and dividing by common Divisors, as 3 and 2; it is found that 10 Feet 6 Inches, will be to 6 Feet 7 Inches, as 3 to 2 nearly: that is, as 15 Miles to 10 Miles.

ble Velocity along the Verge or higheſt Limit of the Atmoſphere; and is generally productive of Wind below.

292. The Elaſticity of the Air muſt likewiſe be brought into the Account, as contributing greatly to its Motion: the Spring of Air always increaſing as the Preſſure encreaſes.

Conſiderable Changes muſt therefore enſue in the inferior Parts of the Atmoſphere.

For as the Effect of the Moon's Attraction is to diminiſh the Weight of the Atmoſphere (tho' its Quantity be increaſed) by elevating the Column of Air in the Line of her Meridian; the Rarefaction of the Air is therefore encreaſed, firſt *at the Top* of the Atmoſphere; afterwards it gradually deſcends to the Bottom, or Surface of the Earth: ſo that the incumbent Weight being diminiſhed, the Air beneath will be greatly *expanded*.

At whatever Height therefore any *Quantity of Vapour* or ſuperior Cloud *reſted*, while the Moon was in her Quarter; it woud *gradually deſcend* at the Approach of the next New or Full: at which Times it woud remain ſuſpended at a Height, where an Expanſion took Place equivalent to the former Expanſion, at the Moon's Quarter: and, if the Height during the Moon's Quarter was only equal to that of common Clouds; ſuch Vapour woud, at the New and Full Moon, *deſcend* in Miſt, Rain, Snow, or Wind.

293. Little Reliance is to be placed, in theſe *Northern* Climates, on the aggregate Weight *(or elaſtic Power)* of the Air, indicated by the Height of the Barometer, near the Times of the New

and

and Full Moons: tho', in general, it will *defcend* about thofe Times.

Thefe Things being fo; it woud be improvident to undertake an aërial Excurfion, either three Days before, or three Days after the Day, either of the New, or Full Moon: the Afcent fhoud be forborne every other Week; at leaft till the Art is a little more advanced.

<small>Proper Days for Afcent.</small>

The two remaining alternate Weeks in each Month, viz. when the Moon is in the Quarters, and the Tide of Air flowing throu' the Atmofphere, is checked, counterbalanced, and equalized, by the lateral Attractions of the Moon and Sun, acting at right Angles, i. e. on different Parts of the Air, pendent on the Earth's Surface;—more fettled and regular Weather may be naturally expected; and particularly freer from the Extremes of *Wind* and *Cold*.

Moreover, as the Almanack, and Ephèmeris (*a*) may be always confulted; the Day fixed on fhoud not be *marked* with Conjunctions of the Planets. (*b*) The Inequality of their united Attractions greatly deranges the Equilibrium of the upper Parts of the Atmofphere; producing fudden Squalls and Gufts of Wind: which, tho' of fhort Continuance, perhaps a few Hours, are inaufpicious to the fuccefsful Inflation and Afcent of a Balloon, during the Infancy of the Science. (See Section 211.)

CHAPTER

(*a*) White's Ephemeris, Page 38, for the Speculum Phenomenorum, or Mirror of the Heavens.

(*b*) See the Book which gives an Account of Walker's Eidouranion.

The *intelligent* Reader will eafily diftinguifh the Effects, attributed to the Planets, viz. their mutual Attractions, owing to natural Caufes only;—from the futile Ravings of judicial Aftrology.

CHAPTER LIII.

ON THE MEANS OF SUSTAINING A BALLOON ABOVE THE SURFACE OF THE WATER, BY A TEMPORARY LOSS OF BALLAST: AND OF RECOVERING THE BALLAST.

Sect. 294. Art. 1. THE two Inconveniencies arising from a *Discharge* of Ballast, while the Balloon is under the *Pressure* of a mediocèanal Column of Air, are,

1. First, lest the Balloon shoud rise too *high:* for by opening the Valve in order to descend; Gas escapes: which is an *actual Loss:* and the Balloon is rendered incapable of supporting its Burden at the same Height, as before.

2. The present Impossibility of resuming the Ballast, in order to *descend*, or *check the Elevation*, on approaching either Shore, or at any other Time.

294. 2. These Inconveniencies are to be remedied by the following Methods.

If *Sand* be the Ballast fixed on; put as much of it into a Bladder by Means of a Tin Funnel, as, when *less* than *half* blown, it will contain, without sinking below the Surface of FRESH *Water*.

Prepare the intended Weight of Ballast, in Bladders, after the same Manner.

Also to EACH Bladder *with Ballast*, tye another Bladder *without Ballast*, half blown.

Tye faft each Set of Bladders, fo prepared, with a *leathern* Thong; the Ends of which may be *left* a few Inches to *fpare*.

The Grapple may remain in the Car.

294. 3. When the Balloon *begins* to defcend over Water; lower out the Cable, by Degrees.

Tye a Pair of Bladders, one of which contains Ballaft, very tight, round the End of the Cable.

Then a fecond Pair, at fuch a Diftance that the intermediate Part of the Cable, will *float*.

Repeat this Procefs, till the proper Effect is obtained; or the whole Ballaft is difcharged.

294. 4. The Car and Balloon may be *hauled* or wound *down* to the Surface of the Water: and the Ballaft refumed, as the Balloon approaches the Shore.

294. 5. If it be found neceffary, the Ballaft may be *difcharged* by cutting the THONGS, *gradually:* or the CABLE, *at once*.

294. 6. If the Wind be *contrary*, and the Weather *moderate*; the Tide, or Stream may, by *Calculation* and *Forefight*, be made to ferve the Purpofe of the Aironaut, in towing the Ballaft which floats on its Surface: and thus checking, or gently drawing the Balloon after it.

294. 7. In fuch Cafes, the Aironaut woud do well in applying his *propulfive* Machinery.

A GENERAL OBSERVATION.

294. 8. To prevent the CAR of the *Balloon* from being drawn out of the Perpendicular, a Circumftance not infrequent; it is neceffary to have fome Contrivance, by which the Cable fhall run throu' a moveable Pulley, on a Swivel, in the

the Center above the Car; and that the Aironaut shall be able *instantly*, by a Screw, or otherways, to fasten the Pulley and Cable so tight, that the Stress shall remain on the Center above the Car, however *forcibly* the Cable may be stretched.

CHAPTER LIIII.

ANOTHER METHOD OF SUSTAINING A BALLOON OVER WATER, WITHOUT LOSS OF GASS, OR OF BALLAST.

Section 295. LET the Ballast consist of that Kind of Rope (wound on a Reel) that is either by Nature or Art, *specifically* lighter than fresh Water: as a *hollow cylindrical* Rope of Silk, in which Corks are thrust: the Silk to be dipped into elastic Varnish, to prevent the Absorption of Water into the Pores: or a common Rope well varnished; or covered over with a cylindric Case of varnished Silk, might answer the same Intention, if Corks or Bladders were tyed at proper Distances: in which Case, the Rope might, at the first Ascent of the Balloon, hang from the Center above the Car, at its full Extent, suppose a Mile or a Mile and half in Length, without the Encumbrance of a Reel.

If Bladders are used; those that hang near the Car shoud not be more than *half blown*.

By the above Expedient; as soon as the Balloon began to decline, from Evaporation of Gass,

Gafs, or Depreffion of the Atmofphere, and the loweft Part of the Rope touched the Water; the Balloon woud continue to levitate, in Proportion to the Quantity of Rope fuftained on the Surface of the Water.

The Aironaut woud move lefs *swift* indeed, but more conveniently; as he woud not be obliged to rife *above* the Wind: but be able to *lower*, and *raise* himfelf at Pleafure: *first*, by pulling up a Part of the Rope into the Car; and having there *made it fast*;

Secondly, by cutting away, as he faw Occafion, the loofe End, and Folds of the Rope fo drawn into the Car with him.

CHAPTER LV.

ON THE NECESSITY OF ASCERTAINING THE PROPER MODES OF DIRECTION, BY DIFFERENT AND FREQUENT EXPERIMENTS.

On the Neceffity of frequent Experiments, in different Modes of Direction.

Section 296. THE Neceffity of making frequent Experiments, in order to prove how far the Balloon is capable of Direction, by different Combinations of the mechanical Powers, is fo apparent; that no Balloon fhoud rife a fecond Time, without the Application of Machinery to that End.

Each Candidate for Fame, as Proprietor of a Balloon for *public Exhibition*, ought to vie in his Pretenfions to a Superiority of Manouvres.

Their

Their respective Performances woud appear in the public Papers; and Decisions be made to the Advantage of the Art.

For it is probable, that by such *Comparison,* chiefly;—the COMPARISON of *experimental Blunders* and *Mistakes,* and not by an Union of Theory and Practice, cemented by liberal Patronage, the Balloon can arrive to any Degree of Perfection, in a Country, which is the Scene of *perpetual Contention:* where the Sum of Life seems devoted but to PARTY; and where the *precious* Time of the GREAT is sunk in Luxury, and their *exalted* Talents lost in the *Labyrinth* of Politics.

297. *To strive against the Stream* is proverbially impossible: and it woud be literally so, to attempt by any Kind of Machinery to force the large Surface of a Balloon, with any Degree of Velocity, against *a Stream of* AIR. (Section 201.)

Ships, which have the Aid of an Element 800 Times *denser* than the AIR, are obliged to wait *in Port,* till the Wind is favourable. But neither is this considered as an Argument against *maritime Navigation:* nor does the *Perfection* of the Balloon require its Ascent in a Storm: tho' the Preference due to the Balloon, on such Occasion, woud be decisive in its Favour: as the latter woud presently surmount the Wind, and *lie to,* in the *calm Air above* it.

Sect. 298. Art. 1. By Wings, or some propulsive Machinery, acting forcibly in a Direction required, and with Ease to the *Operator;* TWO *useful Manouvres* may be attempted, and will frequently be *found successful.*

298. Art. 2.

First Manoeuvre: to secure the Landing in windy Weather.

298. Art. 2. First, To RETARD the Course of the Balloon during its Descent; in such a Manner, as to prevent the Wind from *damaging* the *Machine*, or *snapping the Cable:* and thus to land with Safety, and at the *smallest Distance* BEYOND the Place assigned.

PREPARATORY APPARATUS: and *Signal-Rope.*

298. 3. A *silken*, or other *light* Rope is to be provided: and to run throu' a *snatch Block* fastened to a RUDDER, or to the CAR, as in Crosbie's Balloon (*a*).

Which Rope *alone* woud lessen immediate and unforeseen Danger, by using the Balloon as a Sail, if it actually alighted on the Water.

298. Art. 4. The same Rope being *a Mile*, or *a Mile and Half* in Length; the *Whole*, or a Part of it, might be suffered to run off the Wheel, and, falling on the Surface *below*, in *misty* Weather, woud serve as a Signal to determine whether the Aironaut was over Land, or Water.

Also by winding up his Wheel, he might, if the Weather was moderate, bring himself *down* to the Grapple, which might be so contrived as to *run down* the Rope, and remain at the Bottom, by Means of a Knot, or other Check.

He might also *loose* his Grapple, and *rise* again: or when down; pull the Valve-Cord, and land.

298. 5. With a SECOND short Cable, snatch Block and Grapple, he woud be able to *moor* the Balloon, from which, he might, by procuring the Country People to load the Car with fresh Ballast equal in Weight to himself;—get out, and even leave the Balloon in their Care.

The

(*a*) See London Chronicle, 26th July, 1785.

The Precaution of knowing whether he was over a freſh Water-Lake, (for he might hear the Sea) might be uſeful in miſty and low cloudy Weather by Day, or during the Night; without expending Gaſs in the *exploratory* Deſcent.

298. 6. To facilitate the landing, the *Signal-Rope* may be uſed to the greateſt Advantage, particularly in windy Weather; by *lowering out* a Part, or the Whole, whether a Mile, or Mile and half, ſo that the Grapple may take Effect on the Ground, at the Diſtance of its Length *by Eſtimation, ſhort* of the Place where the Balloon is intended to land.

As ſoon as the Grapple *holds*; it is in the Option of the Aironaut, to tye Parcels of his Ballaſt *looſely* round the Cable, to run downwards along with it.

(For *which Purpoſe*, Iron-Rings with *Spring-Swivels*, which *open* by *Preſſure* of the Fingers, and *ſhut* of themſelves, might anſwer better than the *leathern Thongs*, as the former might be put, in *an Inſtant*, round the Cable, and woud run down *quicker*.)

Theſe Parcels of Ballaſt are to be ſent down, in Succeſſion, till the Balloon has acquired ſuch Degrees of FALSE LEVITY, as will be ſufficient to counteract that Tendency which the Wind will have to *depreſs* the Car of the Balloon forcibly on the Surface, ſo long as it is connected with the Grapple *on the Ground*.

298. 7. When this Point is effected, the Balloon will remain ſuſpended in the Air; and being acted upon by the Wind, will be preſſed into a Direction approaching to an horizontal Line,

Line, in Proportion to the encreafing Power of the Wind.

And here the Neceffity of having the Cable faftened to a Center above the Car, in order to retain its Perpendicularity, is moft evident.

The Aironaut, in this Situation, may venture to wind up the Cable *gradually*, and defcend, to the Grapple.

298. 8. Secondly: When the different Currents of Air, have been tried by Defcent and Afcent of the Pioneer-Balloon *(a)*, and found to be *all* unfavourable; the Aironaut is to *rife* ftill higher, into a Calm, purfue his Courfe horizontally in the BLUE SERENE, by propulfive Machinery: eftimating the Velocity, by the *evident Refiftance* of the half Mile white Flag defcribed in Section 12, 13. and 12, 15. hanging at a proper Diftance *below*, and of that which hangs loofely at the Side of the Car, to fhew a Change in the Direction of the Wind, (then made by a Refiftance of the Air): or he may judge

---

(a) To find the Direction of an upper Current, without the Inconvenience of rifing above the Level which the Aironaut has fixed on.

This the Abbè Bertholon has hinted at, by Means of a fmaller Balloon.

The Dimenfions of which, muft however be fo large; that, allowing for the Evaporation of Gafs, it will *juft* rife with the Weight of a Quantity of Cord, a Mile and half, for Inftance, in Length: and have fufficient Room left within, to admit of the Expanfion of Gafs without Rupture.

The Pioneer-Balloon may be taken up, *empty*, and filled with Gafs neceffarily efcaping from THE MOUTH of the *great Balloon*, when ftationary: and may be fent up with a Cord, faftened to the Center above the Car of the *great Balloon*, to reconnoitre the *fuperior* Currents: or it may be only filled *in Part*; and made to *defcend*, and *difcover* the *lower* Currents.

See " Des Avantages de Ballons, &c. Page 72."

judge of the Velocity and Direction, by the *Flight* of a *Feather*, repeatedly let loose at certain Intervals of Time.

CHAPTER LVI.

NEW MODE OF ASCENT, TO DETERMINE THE INSTANT THE BALLOON IS ARRIVED AT ANY GIVEN HEIGHT: TO MEASURE THE HEIGHTS: AND TO ESTIMATE THE DENSITIES OF THE AIR AT THE GIVEN HEIGHTS.

ALSO, A METHOD OF ASCENDING TO A FIXED BAROMETRIC HEIGHT: THERE TO REMAIN SUSPENDED IN EQUILIBRIO.

Section 299. PREVIOUS to the Ascent, provide a Cord, which shall have sufficient Strength to support twice its own Weight, when so great a Quantity of it is *coiled* together, as, if extended, woud measure half a Mile or a Mile.

Weigh the whole *Coil*, or any Number of Yards, so as to obtain the whole Weight.

Mark the whole Length of the Cord, with different *coloured* Worsted, or otherways, at the Distance of every eight Yards: as a *sounding* Line.

Note the Marks in a Pocket-Book.

These Things being done; give the Balloon, by INFLATION, a Power of Levity *at least* equal to the known Weight of the Cord: which may be easily obtained by throwing into the Car, already *ballasted* and prepared, a Weight equal to the Aironaut, together with that of the *Cord.*

The Cord muft alfo, previous to the Afcent, be rolled upon a Reel, (made faft in the Ground) whofe Diameter fhoud be TWO FEET: each Turn of the Wheel may be called a Yard.

A Barometer with an attached Thermometer fixed in the fame Frame, alfo a fecond or detached Thermometer placed at the Diftance of a Yard from the Frame, fhoud remain upon the Ground during the Inflation.

The fame Apparatus of Barometer with attached and detached Thermometer, fhoud be fufpended in the Car.

The Inftant the Balloon afcends, an Obferver below is to note in a Book the *Point* at which the Quickfilver ftands in each of the THREE Tubes of the lower Apparatus, alfo the Time of Afcent: the Aironaut the fame.

The Rope is, previous to the Afcent, to be tyed to a Center above the Car: and as foon as the Balloon has elevated the Car 100 Yards; the Obfervations, as before, are to be fet down below, and by the Aironaut: and repeated at the Height of each 100 Yards: a Drum to beat; during the Time each Obfervation *below* is *noting down*; and the Balloon not fuffered to rife, till the Drum has ceafed. By fuch repeated *Notice*, and *Silence*; the Aironaut will know the *exact Height*, at which the Balloon is checked in its Elevation: and the *exact Time* during which its Elevation is impeded.

This Procefs is to continue, till the Rope is raifed to its full Length.

At which Inftant a double-barrel Gun is to be

be fired: the exact Time noted *below:* and the Time of hearing the Sound noted above.

These Notes are to be compared at the Aironaut's arrival on Earth.

300. For such *nice* Experiments the Aironaut shoud ascend half an Hour before SUNRISE, or *Sunset*: and the Day chosen by the foregoing Rules.

The Air must be QUITE CALM: but it is not necessary that it shoud be free from Clouds or Mist.

When the Rope is at its full Extent, the Operator *below* is to shorten it, by winding down the Balloon, 100 Yards: the Signals *below*, being repeated, till the Balloon is arrived within 100 Yards of the Ground.

301. While one Observer *below* is writing down the Observation to be made the Instant the Balloon has risen exactly 100 Yards; another Operator is to weigh, by Hand, with Spring Steel-Yards, the Force of Levity already acquired, which is to be noted down by a third Bystander.

To estimate the Densities at different Heights.

This Process is to be repeated at every 100 Yards.

The Levity, it is true, will encrease as the Balloon rises, (probably in a geometric Progression;) (*a*) yet the Cord, by rising with the Balloon, will greatly check it: if, however, it prove

insufficient

(a) As the *Heights* of the Atmosphere encrease in an *arithmetical* Progression; the Densities are said to encrease in a *geometrical* Progression: which is a mathematical and pedantic Mode of Expression.

For *arithmetical* Progression *here* means no more than the Height

insufficient for that Purpose, and, left the Cord shoud be in Danger of breaking; at the second hundred Yards, or, at whatever Height the Levity is found to have encreased 10 Pounds, but is less than 20; a Gun is to be fired as a *fresh* Signal to the Aironaut, who is to scatter away a Bag of Sand-Ballast, (to be put up in Bags of 10 Pounds each;) whenever he hears the Discharge of a Gun.

If the *Cord*, *Rope*, or *Balancer*, be sufficiently strong; there will be no Necessity for the Aironaut to throw out Ballast occasionally; nor for the Observations in the former Part of this Section: the *Densities* will likewise be more easily determined, by the *Weights*; which shew the *Encrease* of Levity and Expansion of the Balloon, at each of the *given* Heights: Allowance being made for the Weight of the *Balance Rope*, raised by the Balloon.

Method of ascending to a fixed *barometric* Height: there to remain suspended *in Equilibrio*.

302. The Aironaut, may, at any Height, marked by looking at the Barometer, when at 24 Inches for Example, or as soon as he finds his Balloon sufficiently expanded, pull up the Rope over a Pulley; or, wind it upon a Reel of two Feet Height of 1, 2, 3, 4, 5, 6, &c. &c. Yards, Fathoms, Roods, or any other equal Interval.

If then at the Height of one Yard, the Balloon has acquired (suppose) the Levity of 1 Pound; then, if this Levity encreases in geometrical Progression; (as twice 1 is 2,) it will, at the Height of 2 Yards, have encreased to 2 Pounds: and, as twice 2 is 4;) it will, at the Height of 3 Yards, have encreased to 4 Pounds: and, as (as twice 4 is 8;) it will, at the Height of 4 Yards, have encreased to 8 Pounds: and, (as twice 8 is 16;) it will, at the Height of 5 Yards, have encreased to 16: and, (as twice 16 is 32;) the Levity will, at the Height of 6 Yards, have encreased to 32 Pounds; and so on, *doubling* the preceding Number; at the Height of each Yard, Fathom, Rood, Mile, &c. &c.

Feet Diameter, within the Car; and continue to do fo; till he finds that the Barometer begins to *rife*, which is a Sign that the Balloon *defcends*, by the additional *Weight* of the Balancer juft brought into the Car: on which, by preconcerted Agreement, he may throw out a WHITE Flag, prepared to hang a Yard below the Car.

On Sight of the Flag, the Perfon at the Reel *below* is to cut the Rope: which Rope, or a Part of it, is to be drawn into the Car.

The Balloon will rife no higher; but remain in *Equilibrio* in the Air, at that Height.

CHAPTER LVII.

ON BALLOONS. THEIR DEFECTS AND FARTHER IMPROVEMENTS.

Section 303. THESE Defects are beft known from the Hiftory: a Detail of which is given to the World in an entertaining, elegant, and fcientific Manner, by a celebrated Writer on other Subjects, *Monf. Faujas de Saint Fond*, in two Volumes, 12mo. for the two laft Years, illuftrated with Engravings by the beft Mafters.

And he promifes a Continuation, or annual Regifter of Experiments and Improvements.

The Title of the Book is, "Defcription des Experiences de la Machine aëroftatique, &c. &c."

304. Mr. Cavallo has favoured the Britifh Nation with a curfory tho' clear Account of the

fame

fame, in his " History of Airoftation:" a Continuation of which it were to be wifhed he woud likewife publifh annually.

305. It might contribute greatly to the Improvement of the Art; if Mr. Faujas woud give Engravings on a large Scale, of the different Machinery, already ufed or invented to direct the Balloon, with their Proportions: particularly the MOULINET of *Blanchard:* as well as that lately tried by Meffrs. Auban and Vallet; whofe Machinery is ftill *more diftinguifhed* and EFFECTUAL.

306. The Titles and Sizes of all ufeful Books written on the Subject, alfo the Places where they are to be had, might likewife be inferted, at the End of each *annual* Volume.

307. The principal Defects of the Britifh Balloons are, in

1. The Conftruction.
2. Production of Gafs.
3. Mode of Direction, and
4. Security of landing.

Firft, Defects of the Conftruction are both in the Form, and Compofition.

The Form ought to be that of a RIGHT (*a*) *Cylinder*, (*b*) by which the *Capacity* is doubled without encreafing the Refiftance: ending above and below, each in a Hemifphere. A cylindrical Trunk, 2 Feet in Diameter, being added to convey the Gafs *into* the Balloon; and fuffer it

to

(*a*) *Whifton's* Tacquet's Euclid. Book XI. Definition of a *right* Cylinder, Art. 3, Page 166.
(*b*) Archimedes's Theorems. Propofition 33, 34; at the End of *Whifton's* Euclid, Page 42.

to escape, when too much expanded in the etherial Regions.

It shoud also be furnished with a Valve, at the Bottom, of equal Diameter with the Trunk: keeping itself Air-tight; and opening outwards by a *given* Resistance, (as that of ten Pounds Troy,) from the inside Gass.

There must be an upper Valve as usual: occasionally to promote a *swift* Descent.

308. The Form will likewise continue to be defective, till an interior Balloon for common Air is adopted, according to the Plan laid down by the ingenious Monsr. Meunier, lately appointed by the French Academy of Sciences at Paris, one of the Commissioners for the Improvement of Airostation.

The Use of which interior Balloon by Compression of the surrounding Gass in the external Balloon, prevents, it is said, the Loss of Ballast and of Gass: two very considerable Advantages.

For the actual Sum total of Gass not being diminished; the Balloon will continue longer in the Air, before an Escape of Gass, throu' the Pores of the Silk, makes it descend.

There will, on the same Account, be less Occasion to take in *meer* Ballast, for the Purpose of throwing it *overboard*, to prevent the Descent.

Therefore an equal Weight of Articles necessary to remain in the Car, may be substituted in Place of the Ballast.

309. Art. 1. And, since it is next *to impossible*, the Atmosphere shoud continue for 24 Hours together, of the *same Density, Weight, and Temperature*; or, in short, without Motion;—the Aironaut

onaut will have a Power of seeking, at *different* Heights, for that Current of Air, or *Wind*, which suits him best: or, in a very few Minutes, to rise above all Currrents; become stationary, and *lie to* in the SERENE, waiting for a *Wind*: which, as before mentioned, he may readily find, by lowering out a Mile of Twine, and his *white* Flag: attending to it, with a small perspective Glass, or Magnifier.

309. 2. Another most *material* Advantage is to be able, in a *high Wind*, to chuse the Spot on which he proposes to alight: or wait for a favourable Opportunity to descend.

To ascertain the Height of the Balloon by a Quadrant. 310. To compute the Height and Distance of the Balloon, by Means of a *white* Flag, or other *visible* Object, suspended from the Car, at a certain Distance below it.

Let the Observer take the Altitude of the Car with a Quadrant: and also the Altitude of the Object or Flag.

Then by a Case in plain Trigonometry; if the Altitude of the Car be by the Quadrant $59° = $ HAC, the Altitude of the Object $55° = $ HAO, and the Length of the Line veered out be 200 Yards, or otherwise $=$ CO.

Then the Complement of HAO $=$ AOH $= 35°$; and the Complement of the Angle HAC $=$ ACH $= 31°$; and the Supplement of OAC $+$ ACO $=$ AOC $= 145°$.

Then, CAO $4°$: CO 200 :: AOC $145°$: AC; and Radius : AC :: CAH $59°$: CH 1409 Yards,

Yards, the Height of the Balloon taken at the Time.

Next, Radius : AC : : ACH 310 : AH 846 Yards, which is the horizontal Diſtance of the Place on the Earth from the Obſerver, over which the Balloon was then ſuſpended.

This Method finds the Height truer than the Barometer, and with fewer Circumſtances of Confuſion.

And if the Balloon Art coud be perfected, ſo as to make them ſtationary at any Height; this Circumſtance woud afford excellent Opportunities of proving the Heights by the Barometer: beſides which, the Diſtance alſo has been obtained : a Point not before attempted. *(a)*

CHAPTER LVIII.

OF THE AIR-BOTTLE BALLOON.

Section 311. TILL the Particulars of Meunier's Invention are made public, *(b)* an additional *Air-tight* Balloon, or Air Bottle, at leaſt 15 Feet in Diameter, of a *globular* Form, appended below the Car, and furniſhed with a *Condenſer*, to be worked by *pulling upwards*, or, as the Bellows of an Organ, by the alternate Motion of the Feet of the Aironaut, ſtanding upright in the Car, may be uſed inſtead of the interior Balloon; to keep the *great Balloon*

(a) Inſerted in the Cheſter Chronicle, Sept. 30, 1785.
(b) The Writer not having yet been able to procure it from the London Bookſellers.

at a *given* Height: and confequently prevent the Aironaut *from rifing too high:* to atchieve which Purpofe, during the *firft Afcent*; a Rope or Balancer may be ufed, a Mile and half long, faftened to the Car, and rifing with the Balloon, (to *check* its Power of *Afcent,*) till an Equilibrium is produced: at which Inftant, on Sight of the *white* Flag from the Car, the Balance-Rope is to be cut, by the Operator *below.* (Section 302.)

If the Aironaut perceives by the Rife of the *Barometer*, that the Balloon defcends; he may throw out a *little* Ballaft, (perhaps a Pound or two), and then wind up his Balancer, or fuffer it to remain at any Length, at his Option.

312. By keeping the Balloon at a given Height *only*; no Gafs is expended in preventing the neceffary Tendency of Balloons to a perpetual Elevation: alfo, during the felf Defcent of the Balloon; by opening the Air-Bottle, the Aironaut will fupercede the Neceffity of throwing out Ballaft, for a Re-afcent.

313. The Air-Bottle-Balloon fhoud be covered by a ftrong *light* Net, of a Dimenfion rather lefs than the Bottle, which will hinder it from burfting: the Refiftence of the *condenfed* Air within, being then chiefly on the Net, and but little on the Bottle.

The Net may be made of Silk and Cotton Thread; left the Mefhes, by the Preffure of the Knots, fhoud eat into the Bottle.

CHAPTER

CHAPTER LIX.

SUPERIORITY OF THE AIR-BOTTLE TO AN INTERIOR BALLOON.

Section 314. THE Air-Bottle can be attended with no Sort of Danger. For, if it burst; the only Effect is to raise the Balloon: which is made to descend, at Pleasure, by opening either the *lower* or upper Valve.

Whereas an interior Balloon condensed with common Air, presses against the surrounding exterior Gass: and the Gass, against the INSIDE of the *great Balloon*, when the latter is in an elevated and rarefied Atmosphere; which Atmosphere, in Proportion to its Height, makes *less* Resistance to the *Outside* of the great Balloon: and thereby encreases its Tendency to a Rupture.

By the Application of the Air-Bottle, which will be to a Balloon, what an Air-Bladder, or *Swim* is to a Fish; a **concomitant** Advantage is derivable.

For the common Balloon and Air-Bottle, which may be called A DOUBLE BALLOON, will, in their *present imperfect* State, be able to remain a Day, or perhaps a Couple of Days in the Air: there being no Loss of Gass: unless by Evaporation, throu' the Pores of the Silk.

And this Advantage of *a double Balloon* may be effected with little EXPENCE (except that of a complete Net) to the different Proprietors, who may make alternate Voyages, with the Balloons *thus* united: one being inflated with Gaſs; the other occaſionally with three or more Atmoſpheres of common Air *condenſed*.

CHAPTER LX.

HINTS FOR THE DIRECTION OF THE BALLOON.

Sect. 315. Art. 1. IN the London Chronicle, from the 20th to the 22d of Auguſt, 1785, is a Letter from Bury, containing an Account of Mr. Poole's Balloon, with the following Circumſtance, viz. " It was found neceſſary, before the Balloon was liberated, to cut away the Wings, intended to act as Sails, which had been conſtructed by an ingenious Piedmonteſe, patronized by LORD ORFORD, and which it was ſuppoſed, woud have contributed *to facilitate the Direction of the* Balloon, but were found *greatly to retard the Celerity* of its Motion."

Now if any Credit can be given to Newſpaper Accounts, (that of the Beccles Balloon being an entire Fable,) it is to be lamented that the Wings were cut away for the Reaſon aſſigned: as it ſeems the only one that coud properly be offered for applying them.

315. 2. Balloons already riſe like a Rocket, and preſs forward almoſt with the Celerity of the Wind: it is therefore evident, that theſe Celerities

ties muft be *greatly retarded*, in order *to facilitate the Direction :* and confequently that the Wings bid fair to have anfwered the Intention of their ingenious Projector. And why precipitately cut them away, before the Balloon was left to the Pleafure of the Winds? fince no regular or fafe Manouvres ought to have been attempted, till that Time.

There appears to have been much the fame Reafon for rejecting the Piedmontefe Wings, that there was for condemning the ufe of a Parafhute, to which a Dog being appended was killed in the Defcent: becaufe the Parafhute was not let loofe at a fufficient Height, nor was it properly diftended.

315. 3. It feems, that as the Wings had *greatly* IMPEDED the Balloon; a certain *Addition* to them might have *nearly* STOPPED it in the Air.

For the Balloon having once acquired an uniform Motion, by encreafing the Surface of the refifting Body, or Wings, the Balloon may be retarded to a certain Point. But the Refiftence encreafing woud raife the refifting (*a*) Body above its Power of Action, and therefore, in Fact, leffen it; by which Means the Balloon woud continue to be propelled in the Direction of the Wind, with a Force equal to that Diminution.

Suppofe, for Inftance, that, inftead of the half Mile Flag, which evidently checked the progreffive Motion of the Balloon (Section 70) a larger fquare Surface, of varnifhed Silk, or a triangular Latteen Sail (like the Ἀρτεμων of Le Roi (*b*))

was

(*a*) See Chambers's Dictionary under the Article RESISTENCE.

(*b*) See his " Navires des Anciens."

was substituted, and kept stretched, by a hollow Cane, or Yard. *(c)*

315. 4. Also, that by Means of a Fan or small Oar, acting as a Rudder, to be folded and taken back into the Car at Pleasure, the Balloon was compelled to move with a given Side foremost; that the Sail was let down below the Car, by strong silken Cords fastened to each Angle; and lastly, that leaden Weights, (each weighing an Ounce Averdupoise when widely perforated, and put throu' the Ends of each Cord before it is fastened to the Car), be let down to each Angle; occasionally encreasing the Weights (or Sail) in Proportion to the Wind; which relative Weights (or Sail) will best be determined by repeated Experiments; will not such an Apparatus or Anemometer-Sail, acting as a Vis Inertiæ nearly at right Angles against the Force of the Wind, check the Balloon; till the encreasing Resistence raising the Sail upwards towards the Horizon diminishes its Power of Action? With this Sail therefore, which requires little Attention; and with the Assistance of Wings moved by Levers, pressed alternately downwards as the Bellows of an Organ, by the Feet of the Aironaut and mere Weight of his Body, standing upright near the Center of the Car; the Balloon may probably be, in some Respect, subject to Direction, and move obliquely against the Wind, or with Force in a Calm.

The Balloon and Anemòmeter-Sail, like the Earth

(c) See " Gordon's Principles of Naval Architecture."
Also the Balzaes and Guaraes, in Ullòa's Voyage to America, Book 4, Chapter 9, Vol. 1, Page 183.

Earth and Moon will turn on their common Center of Gravity.

315. 5. It is poſſible to erect a light hollow Maſt throu' the Car, and throu' the Balloon, by Means of a cylindrical Tube of varniſhed Silk, extending from Top to Bottom, in order to ſuſtain the Balloon in an upright Situation, and make it keep Pace with the Car, when the latter is propelled by the Wings. The Maſt ſhoud be covered with ſoft Cotton, to leſſen the Roughneſs of the Friction. It may alſo contain within it, another ſlenderer hollow Maſt, after the Manner of a Cane Fiſh-Rod; either to be lowered out, and placed horizontally acroſs or below the Car, to ſerve as a Guard for the Bottom of the Anemòmeter-Sail; or to be let down to any Depth occaſionally: and other Sails connected, by the uſual wooden Rings, and kept tight by Cords running throu' Blocks faſtened to any Part of *the equatorial Hoop*, as uſed at firſt, by the *gallant Admiral of the Air* BLANCHARD, and afterwards too precipitately rejected; ſince, in Caſe of a Rupture of Gaſs throu' the upper Hemiſphere of the Balloon; the equatorial Hoop preſerves the Paraſhute complete: and for Want of which Hoop, young Arnold had certainly loſt his Life, if the Water of the Thames had not broke his Fall.

During the Deſcent of the Balloon, the Sails are to be taken in, and the lower Maſt projected into its Socket.

315. 6. Different Trials may be repeatedly made: the Effects of which, whether evidently uſeful or *apparently otherwiſe*, being carefully recorded

corded and regularly publifhed *in Detail*, may afford Data for the Profecution of further Difcoveries, and lay the Foundation for a rational Superftructure of *airoftatic Navigation*.

On the Manner in which the Wind, Anemòmeter, and propulfive Machinery will probably operate on the Balloon.

Sect. 316. Art. 1. By adding Weights, and encreafing the Surface of Anemòmeter-Sails; the Vis Inertiæ will become fo powerful in the Direction of the refifting Medium of the Air; that the Wind in the oppofite Direction will force the Balloon out of its Vertical, and incline it to the Horizon. The Car will be a Fulcrum Axis or Center of Motion: on an imaginary Point of which, as on a Pivot, the Balloon and Sails will turn oppofite Ways, balancing each other in every Situation.

316. 2. The Balloon muft therefore be brought back into the Vertical by a counter Exertion of the Wings: to which the Vis Inertiæ muft allways be made to bear a juft Proportion.

The Declination of the Balloon is the only Inconvenience forefeen to refult from an Anemòmeter too large, or too heavily laden: and it is inftantly remedied by flacking the Sail.

One Thing ftill remains to be mentioned.

317. Balloons *durably* Air-tight, and terminating in a *Hemifphere* above, (Section 307); ought to have their Dimenfions fuch, that there fhoud be no Occafion for more than their upper Hemifphere to be inflated. Under which Form, they may with Eafe and Safety be pitched as Tents on the Ground; by Cords faftened at equal Diftances to the equatorial Hoop; and on Occafion by the Aironaut himfelf, while in the Car: who may be provided with

Iron

Iron Ring Stakes barbed, and faftened or ready to be faftened to each Balloon-Cord: and, as foon as the Balloon is moored by the Anchor, Grapple, and fnatch Block, (Section 298, 3) with a light Axe drive down the Stakes round the Car, and regulate them when he alights from it, on the Ground.

CHAPTER LXI.

HINT FOR A VANE-SAIL TO PREVENT THE BALLOON FROM TURNING ROUND, WHILE THE WIND CONTINUES STEADY.

Section 318. TO the Block-Pulley in the equatorial Hoop, hoift a Sail, *Hint for a Vane-Sail.* whofe Shape is as follows.

From the equatorial Hoop, let fall a Perpendicular: and from the loweft circular Point in the Circumference of the Balloon, draw a Tangent, or horizontal Line, till it meet the former: thefe Lines, together with that Part of the Circumference intercepted between them, in the Points where they touch the Circle, forms a Space, which is the Shape fought.

The Sail may be kept fteady by a hollow Cane or Bowfprit thruft out from the Car, and made faft with the ufual Tackling.

319. Hint for an Umbrella-Pendulum or Valve-Swing, to project the Balloon in a Calm in the ethereal Regions, above the Station of Clouds;

where

where the Refiftance from the Air is much lefs than at the Surface of the Earth.

Hint for a Valve-Swing to project the Balloon in a calm and elevated Atmofphere.

Let the Car of the Balloon be perforated fo as to admit a light Gordon Maft, or Pole 18 or 20 Feet long, perpendicularly throu' it. (315, 3.)

At the Diftance of five Feet from the upper End of the Pole, a light hollow cylindric Tube of Iron, one Foot long, as a Bolt, fhoud be put throu' it, at right Angles: fo as to play fmoothly in two Iron Bends, fixed in the Car; one Bend fo far moveable, as to rife with a Hinge to admit the End of the Bolt; the other Part of the Bend to be perforated: throu' which a hollow Staple is to be faftened, with a fpring Cotterel chained: this Apparatus will prevent the Pole from turning round.

Two light Frames of Wood, of a parallelogrammic Form, each twelve Feet by fix, and covered with varnifhed Silk, are to be hooked, one on each of the oppofite Sides of the Pole, from its lower End upwards; the Frames to be moveable in fuch a Manner, that on preffing the Pole one Way on the Axis or Bolt, the Frames fhall lie clofe; but on recovering the Preffure, the Frames fhall expand and open, fo as to form an obtufe Angle with each other, or to lie almoft in the fame Plane, when the Recovery is made brifkly, and with a Degree of Strength.

A Handle of Wood, the fame Size with the Bolt, may be faftened throu' the Subftance of the Pole near its upper End.

The Operator is to ftand in the Car, and work the Pole backwards and forwards, which will give

give a progressive Motion to the Balloon in a Calm.

This Method may possibly prove more effectual than the Umbrella-Wheels, on an horizontal Axis, of Monsf. Carra (*a*); as the Umbrella-Pendulum is easily unrigged, removed, and brought into the Car, in Case of a Whirlwind; by Means of a *circular* Rope fastened to the Axis or Bolt, one End being in the Car, and the other put throu' the Aperture at the Bottom, and brought up from the Outside again into the Car.

The Umbrella-Pendulum may be made to turn round horizontally on the Bolt; the Ends of the Bolt being fastened under a circular hinged Socket, or Groove, of Iron.

CHAPTER LXII.

DEFECTS, IN THE COMPOSITION FOR BALLOONS, REMEDIED.

ALSO ON THE COCHUC-VARNISH.

Section 320. BALLOONS are defective in the Composition for *the Varnish*; which, till lately, was incapable of rendering the Balloon completely and *durably* Air-tight.

321. It

(*a*) Monsf. Carra proposed to ascend with two Balloons. One, a seventh Part less than the other, is to be connected by a Rope, throu' a Pulley fixed in the equatorial Hoop of the great Balloon, to a Reel in the Center of the Car: in descending, the Reel is to be unwound: the great Balloon and Car will therefore descend, while the small Balloon remains in the Air. The Scheme is certainly practicable. See the Cut in the London Magazine for June, 1784.

321. It was sometime ago reported at Paris, that Mr. Dutourny de Villiere had undertaken to construct a Balloon so truly *impèrmeable*, that he woud warrant the Duration of it, for *several Weeks* in the Air.

And it is *since* known that this *Desideratum* of the Art has been effected, in the Composition for the celebrated Balloon of Messrs. Auban and Vallet, FIRST made subject to Direction.

322. Mr. Berniard, a French Chymist, has made curious tho' unsuccessful Experiments, in order to melt the cochuc or elastic Bottle; as may be seen in the 17th Volume of the " Journal de Physique."

Mr. Faujas and others made similar Trials.

323. The Writer, unacquainted with what had *then* been done in this Matter, coud not help remarking the striking Properties of the *Cochuc* in its present Form, to answer every Intention of the best Varnish, if its Price was lower;—viz. *compact, pliant, unadhesive,* and *unalterable by Weather*;—if it coud be dissolved, and afterwards made to recover its present UNADHESIVE Form: an Art in which the East and West-Indians are still *our Masters.*

He has, however, after expensive Trials and Combinations, been able to reduce it into a *limpid Liquor.*

As it may prove a useful Ingredient for *Air-tight* Varnish; the Secret he now discovers to the World: and it is merely this.

324. " Take any Quantity of the Cochuc, as two Ounces Averdupois: cut it into small Bits, with a Pair of Scissars.

Put

Put a strong Iron-Ladle (such as Plumbers or Glaziers melt their *Lead* in) over a common Pit-Coal or other Fire.

The Fire must be gentle, glowing, and *without* Smoke.

When the Ladle is hot, much below a RED *Heat*; put a single Bit into the Ladle.

If *black* Smoke issues, it will presently *flame*, and disappear: or it will evaporate without Flame: the Ladle is *then* too hot.

When the Ladle is less hot, put in a second Bit, which will produce a WHITE *Smoke*.

This WHITE *Smoke* will continue during the Operation, and evaporate the Cochuc: therefore no Time is to be lost: but little Bits are to be put in, a few at a Time, till the whole are melted. It shoud be continually and gently stirred with an Iron or Brass Spoon.

The Instant the Smoke changes from *white* to BLACK, take off the Ladle; or the whole will break out into a violent Flame, and be spoiled or lost.

(Care must be taken that *no Water* be added: a few Drops only of which, woud—on Account of its superior *specific Gravity*, for the Cochuc swims in Water—make it boil over furiously, with great Noise.)

At this Period of the Process; two Pounds, or one Quart of the BEST DRYING-OIL, (or even of *raw* Linseed-Oil, which, together with a few Drops of Neat's-Foot-Oil, must have stood a Month, or not so long, on a Lump of Quick-Lime, to make it more or less DRYING)—being poured off the Lime-Lees; is to be put into the

melted

melted Cochuc, and ftirred till hot: and the whole poured into a glazed Veffel, throu' a coarfe Gauze, or fine Sieve.

When fettled and clear, which will be in a few Minutes; it is fit for Ufe, either hot or cold.

The Silk fhoud be ftretched all Ways horizontally, by Pins or Tenter-Hooks, on Frames; which Frames, the greater they are in Length, the better: and the Varnifh poured on COLD, in *hot* Weather; and HOT, in *cold* Weather.

It is *perhaps* beft, always to lay it on, when *cold*.

The Art of laying it on properly, confifts in making NO INTESTINE Motion in the Varnifh, which woud create minute Bubbles. Therefore Brufhes of every Kind are improper.

Each Bubble breaks in drying, and forms a fmall Hole, throu' which the *Air* will *tranfpire*.

CHAPTER LXIII.

ON VARNISHES, CONTINUED.

Section 325. TO thofe, who are unacquainted with the Principles of Chemiftry, or the Books which teach it; and yet are defirous to make Experiments, which may throw frefh Light on this curious and ufeful Art, when applied to Varnifhes for Umbrellas or Balloons; the following detached Notes are recommended: which were communicated to the Author by *different* Artifts; each *eminent* in his Profeffion.

326. To

326. To make copal Varnish.

Procure some bluish Flemish alcaline Ashes, (an Ounce suppose): pound them *very fine*, and lay them before the Fire, till they become HOT and DRY.

Put them, while hot and dry, into Oil of Turpentine, (a Pint or Pound for Instance): or, into the same Quantity of Spirits of Wine.

For by Means of the Alcaly, *(a)* all the Water invisibly contained in the Oil or Spirits will be absorbed, and leave the Oil or Spirits, ALCOHOL, that is, quite pure, and highly rectified: which Process is called *alcalizing* the Turpentine, or Spirits.

Put the Turpentine or Spirits so alcalized, into a Copper Vessel, with half an Ounce of YELLOW COPAL *finely* pounded and sifted.

Stir it, and the Copal will soon melt.

N. B. If you alcalize the Spirit of Turpentine, when the Copal is dissolving, add a little Spirit of Wine: and if you alcalize the Spirit of Wine, when the Copal is dissolving, add a little Spirit of Turpentine.

The SEDIMENT of the Varnish will dry on the Silk, in a few Hours.

The thicker the Varnish, the sooner it dries.

327. Article 1. To make an excellent THIN Varnish.

To one Quart of *cold raw* Linseed-Oil poured off from the Lees made by a Lump of *unslacked* Lime on which the Oil has stood, ten or eight Days, at the least, in order to communicate a drying Quality: (or on *brown Umber* burnt and pounded,

(a) See " Lewis's Commerce of the Arts."

pounded, which will have the like Effect:)—add half an Ounce of Litharge.

Boil them for half an Hour.

Then add half an Ounce of *the Copal Varnish*.

327. 2. While the Ingredients are on the Fire, in a Copper Vessel; put in one Ounce of Chio Turpentine, or common Rezin: and a few Drops of NEAT'S-FOOT-OIL: and stir the whole with a Knife, or any clean Thing.

When *cold*, it is ready for Use.

327. 3. The Neat's-Foot-Oil prevents the Varnish from being sticky, or adhèsive: and may be put into the Linseed-Oil, at the same Time with the Lime, or burnt Umber.

327. 4. To make the above Varnish *transparent*, or *white*; use Mastic and Copal: to make it *brown*, use Seed or Shell-Lac, and *browner still*, use *pounded burnt* Umber.

327. 5. *Rezin*, or *Chio Turpentine* may be added, till the Varnish has obtained the desired *Thickness*.

327. 6. It must likewise be observed, that *Litharge* rots the Silk: therefore Trials must be made without the Use of Litharge.

327. 7. The *longer* the raw Linseed-Oil remains on the unslacked Lime, or Umber, the *sooner* will the Oil dry, after it is used.

If some Months; so much the better. Such Varnish will *set*, i. e. will not run, but keep its Place on the Silk, in four Hours.

The Silk may then be turned, and varnished on the other Side.

328. ON GUM MASTIC, SANDARAC, SEED-LAC, SHELL-LAC, AND COPAL.

328. 1. Gum *Mastic* dissolves, *without pounding,*

ing, by adding a few Drops of Oil of Vitriol: so do Gum *Sandarac*, and Gum *Copal*, when finely pounded and sifted.

328. 2. Gum *Sandarac*, and Gum *Mastic* are great Driers of themselves: and may be substituted for Litharge.

328. 3. The Mastic dissolved in the Oil of Vitriol, gives a *sweet* Smell to the Varnish.

328. 4. Sandarac will soon grow *dusk* in the Fire: it melts into a transparent Liquor.

328. 5. Sandarac, Seed-Lac, and Shell-Lac, must be finely pounded and sifted, before they are used.

329. The Author having examined different Kinds of varnished Silks, in different Places, does, from their Excellence, recommend those made by *Fawkner*, Umbrella-Maker, Alport-Street, Manchester; a Person wholly unknown to him, but from the Merit of the Work: which consists not only in the Varnish itself; but in the peculiar Method of *applying* it, which the Author *is not at Liberty to make public*.

Fawkner can warrant his Silk *Air-tight*; *soft* and *unadhesive*; durable, and *unalterable* by that Excess of Heat and Cold, to which the Balloon is, at the same Time, subject; viz. *internally*, to the hot depredating and caustic Fumes, rising with the Gass: and *externally*, to the *Sun*, *Wet*, *Frost*, and *Drought*.

CHAPTER LXIV.

HINTS ON IMPROVEMENT OF THE MACHINERY.

Section 330. IN order to make Improvements of the Balloon still more rapid and general; the Society for the Encouragement of Arts, who have given no particular Encouragement, in Imitation of that at Lyons, to the much-wished-for Art of directing the Balloon;—might offer a Premium for different Inventions of a *propulsive Machinery*, the Models of which are to be made at the Expence of the Society, within a certain limited Sum: and, without condemning what cannot be known unless by repeated Trials,—give Encouragement for such Trials: the Models to remain with the Society for public Exhibition.

331. Also, Figures and Explanations of such Machinery as have been tried, viz. the Fly or Moulinet of Blanchard; and of those which have not succeeded for Want of Trial; might be sent by the Inventors, in order to perpetuate the Invention, either to the *Society of Arts*; or to the Editors of creditable Magazines, who woud be glad of such ingenious Acquisitions, as it woud be a Means of procuring Purchasers, and circulate the Knowledge of this *gigantic* Infant Science.

Improvement woud then go on apace, and in a Chain: each Labourer forging and finishing his respective Link.

Whereas at present every one is obliged to find his own Materials, sink the Foundation, raise and finish the Building. And hence so little Work is done, worthy the Inspection of a skilful Architect.

CHAPTER LXV.

ON THE UTILITY OF BALLOONS:
AN INTRODUCTORY CHAPTER.

Sect. 332. Art. 1. IT seems a favourite Question, among those who take a Pleasure in objecting to every Thing they neither do nor will understand, to ask, " Of what Use can these Balloons be made?" and without waiting for an Answer, to say—" they pick the Pockets of the Public, risque the Lives of the Incautious, encourage Mobbing and Sharpers, and terrify all the World." These trite Reasonings are all very true, but little to the Purpose: the Effects above described being merely those arising from Novelty. If, says one in an inferior Station; " they coud convert Balloons into common Stage Waggons; Goods might be carried with the greater Expedition:" or, " into Stage Coaches," says another: or, " into Mail Coaches" says Palmer; " it woud be certainly very clever, as I have the Patent:"—" or into comfortable Carriages to step in out of THE WINDOW, at a Moment's Notice; that woud be something," cries a Nobleman: " it woud *save* one a Couple of Sets of Horses, and woud eat Nothing: one might ride one's own Balloon Matches, from one's Window to Newmarket, and from Newmarket to TOWN; dress for Court as we *do*, and make *Nothing* of it."

Such are the different Ideas annexed by different Ranks of Men, to the Word UTILITY when applied to Balloons.

332. 2. For once let the feeble Voice of a French Philofopher be heard, the Abbée Bertholon: who may perhaps affert that all this is not impoffible.

A Series of Experiments only can determine: and let the following Remarks ferve as an Introduction to his Opinions.

332. 3. It is certain that the Progrefs already made in the Improvement of Balloons, fince their Invention only three Years ago, is far fuperior to the Acquirements in every other Art.

The Antients knew, that excited Amber attracted Straws, and certain other light Subftances: but medical Electricity, and a Prefervative from Lightening, were notwithftanding referved for the Moderns.

They likewife attended to fome ftriking Effects of the natural Loadftone: but were totally unacquainted with the artificial Magnet, and the amazing Powers conferrable by it in the Diforders of the Imagination: nor did they know the Polarity of its Needle, or Application of it in the Compafs.

They had not combined Nitre and Sulphur with Charcoal: much lefs had they changed the Mode of War into Science, by eftablifhing Founderies for Cannon, and the Study of Tactics. Yet fome Nations with a Knowledge of the Moderns, as the Chinefe, have not improved, even in the Conftruction of their Veffels, according to the European Manner; continuing ftill in practical Ignorance.

Nor have other Indians improved in Proportion

tion to the Opportunities of Inftruction in feveral Arts.

Thofe of America, for Example, who continue to hunt, fifh, and fcalp: neglecting the Plough, and other Arts of Property and Peace.

332. 4. And thus it has been with the Britifh Nation on the Subject of Airoftation.

Cavendifh, Prieftley, and others, had produced inflammable Air, weighed, and found it lighter than common Air: and all that had feen a bright Fire might conclude, if they reafoned at all, that hot Air was lighter than cold.

Yet if Montgolfier had not made, ON A LARGE SCALE the Application of hot Air, in a Bag open at the Bottom, and properly poifed; Charles and Roberts woud probably not have thought of applying the Gafs of Cavendifh: and Mankind woud not *yet* have foared into the etherial Regions.

332. 5. In this the French are ftill before the Englifh, and will continue fo to be, without a laudable and unlooked-for Emulation in the latter. That the former admire Liberty, Montefquieu's "Spirit of Laws" may determine; but they are not *addicted* to Politics. Their Nobility are endowed with a liberal and enterprizing Spirit. They join and patronize Men of Genius and Talents in the Cultivation of the Arts, and Improvement of every Kind of experimental Knowledge. Their Pleafure confifts in a national Ambition to excel.

They have Leifure, and are fober.

Half that Time which Men of Fortune in France dedicate to Tafte, Invention, and Refinement;

ment; Britons spend among the Beasts and Birds: the other half, at the Bottle, and in political Cabals.

Present Profit is almost the sole Motive for Excellence in Great-Britain: and Experiments(a) not made with that View, are seldom repeated; are overlooked and forgotten.

CHAPTER LXVI.

ON THE UTILITY OF BALLOONS.

Section 333. THE Balloon opens a new and unlimited Field for Philosophical Discoveries.

334. The many curious and interesting Conjectures which Monſ. de Luc (before the Invention of Balloons) throws out, in the Course of 4 large Volumes, on the Subject and Qualities of the Atmosphere; may now be determined by actual Trial.

335. The Abbèe Bertholon wrote in 1784: and has particularly mentioned the following Points, as capable of ample Investigation, and Discussion.

Sect. 336. Art. 1. *The Temperature of the Air at different Heights.*

Which will determine whether the Atmosphere be *practically Navigable*, at all Times and Places.

306. 2. *The*

(a) See Prieſtley's numerous Experiments: and that Library of *curious Inveſtigation*, the Philoſophical Tranſactions.

336. 2. *The dissolvent Power of the Air by Means of an Atmometer for Evaporation.*

Probably the Height may be determined, to which Clouds commonly ascend in order to find the proper horizontal Level, in which Balloons can move with the greatest Ease, Safety, and Expedition.

336. 3. *Variations of the Barometer.*

This will ascertain the exact Height, without Mensuration.

336. 4. *The* DENSITIES *at different Heights.*

A principal Object in de Luc's abstruse and scientific Researches: not only useful but necessary to determine the Laws of Refraction; without which, Astronomy, and consequently NAVIGATION, must remain defective.

336. 5. *The different Effects of Tastes, and Odors, at different Heights: Experiments on Plants and Animals: also of* SOUND.(a)

These may produce new and salutary Effects on the human Body: and determine how far a Change from hot, putrid, and impure, to cool pure Air, impregnated with the invigorating aërial Acid, may contribute, without the Aid of Drugs, to the Recovery of the Sick, and Invalid: or promote Longevity.

336. 6. *The Direction and Velocity of the Wind.*

The different Currents and their different Heights, the Limitation of each Stratum of Wind, together with their different Temperatures

---

(a) And *Magnitude* of distant Objects.
Bacon says that Objects are more *visible* in an East Wind, and Sounds more *audible* in a West Wind; being heard at a *greater* Distance. " Historia Ventorum, P. 37, Art. 31."

tures at the same Time, will point out the proper Paths for the Balloon to move in, at all Times, and *possibly* without the Necessity of accurate Direction: the Mode of Ascent and Descent being *already* known, and proper Instructions given for a secure Landing.

336. 7. *Electricity of the Air*, METEORS.

This may lead to the Birth Place of Lightening, and Methods how to avoid its Effects in the Air. Tho' it be already known, that little Danger is to be apprehended, on Account of the mutual Repellency between the electric Fluid, inflammable Gass, and oiled Silk.

The Irides, the Coronaes, Haloes, and other Phenomena of Colours: the Generation and Solution of which may be investigated on the Spot.

336. 8. *Geography may become a new Science.*

336. 9. *Use of the Balloon for Signals in the calm Air, above Molestation; above Winds still blowing below: to discover the Positions of an Army, or Navy.*(a)

336. 10. *To throw principal Men into a Town: and convey others out of it.*

336. 11. With the Montgolfier Balloon, to try Experiments on Light, and Fire: to transport great Weights: raise them out of the Water: draw up Piles, raise Trees, Vessels, &c.

336. 12. The Parashute to secure a Man from too precipitate a Fall, is to be 5 Yards in Diameter, when extended: the Man,—weighing 140 Pounds, and the Parashute weighing 10 Pounds, with a Surface of 150 square Feet,—woud, in that Case,

---

(a) See Le Roi's Uses of the airostatic Globe *at Sea*, in his "Navires des Anciens, Page 225."

ON THE FORM AND DIRECTION OF BALLOONS. 265

Cafe, feel no greater Shock than if he had fallen from the Height of six Feet.

336. 13. *The Compaſs and its Variations: alſo the different Branches in Aſtronomy.*

His Hints on the Direction of the Machine are ingenious.

337. 1. Wheels furniſhed with Wings.

337. 2. Imitations of the Form and Motions of Fiſh. (*a*)

337. 3. Veſſels to condenſe Air, as the Bladders of Fiſh.

337. 4. Wind-Guns, Wind-Fountains.

337. 5. Elopile and Vapour Steam.

337. 6. Contrary Currents at different Heights: Proof of.

337. 7. New Hints for Balloons to be raiſed by Steam.

337. 8. Monſ. Gouan's Invention to go THREE HUNDRED MILES A DAY IN A CALM.

338. The general Uſe to which Balloons ſeem capable of being applied, with the Aſſiſtance of propulſive Machinery, in the Calm which exiſts

M m above

(*a*) The *natural Figure* of the *Diodon-Globe-Fiſh*, a coloured Print of which is given in " Martyn's new and elegant Dictionary of natural Hiſtory:" where it is deſcribed as follows: " The Form of the Body is uſually oblong: but when the Creature is alarmed, it poſſeſſes the Power of *inflating* its Belly to a globular Shape of great Size;"—ſeems to furniſh a Hint for the proper Figure of a Balloon, when the Art is more improved.

The Balloon, as far as it is meant to reſemble the upper Part of the Fiſh, is to be made ſtiff, with Paſteboard or *Papier-mâché* varniſhed; for, being ſtrong, and in a permanent Form, it is more capable of continuing Air-tight: the lower Parts being *flaccid*, will be inflated, as the Balloon riſes, and deflated during the Deſcent.

Rowers, and propulſive Machinery, are to be fixed within the Fiſh, in Place of the Fins: and Goods of GREATER Weight placed in a covered Car below: the Air-Bottle-Balloon being fixed between both.

above the Level of a CONTRARY Wind; is that of a common Vehicle, not subject to the Inconvenience of Roads and Inns, between distant Places and Countries, for Passengers, properly accommodated in a Boat-shaped covered Car, furnished with Provisions, and occasional Siberian Cloathing: the Car to be surrounded with, and resting on Bladders, one *fourth blown*, and having each a few Drops of Water within, to keep them moist and elastic;—to prevent an *accidental* Shock in alighting on Land; and from sinking, if on Water.

Such a Conveyance (the Balloon being once made *Air-tight*, and furnished with an *Air-Bottle* to ascend and descend *without Loss* of Gass) is ready at all Seasons and Times: both Night and Day: for, as the Aironauts will enjoy continual Sunshine without a Cloud, from his Rising to his Setting: so, during the Night, the Light of the STARS, always intercepted in their Passage to the Earth by Clouds or thick Vapours, will be greatly augmented, when above both: besides the probable Increase of Light *reflected* from the upper Fields of white Clouds shone on continually by the different Planets and Constellations: all which will afford an Illumination equal, if not greater, than that of a cloudless frosty Night, when the Ground is covered with Snow.

And such Light will be sufficient to read or write by: also to examine the *Barometer*, (a) in order to know the *Height* and Level of the Balloon above the Surface of the Earth: and the COMPASS for Direction.

If

(a) And by *Kunckel*'s or *Canton*'s Phosphorus. See "Priestley's History of LIGHT. Pages 585, 370."

If Aironauts propofe to afcend by Night, and in the Moon's Quarters; obferving likewife the Precautions already given; it may be proper alfo to confult and take with them the Ephèmeris, in order to know the Time when the Moon rifes, and alfo when fhe is at the higheft, i. e. in the South, or has remained about half her Time above the Horizon.

The plaineft Points, on which not only the Succefs of an Excurfion, but the Lives of Aironauts may depend, are too frequently neglected, as unimportant and trivial.

CHAPTER LXVII.

THE PROCESS OF INFLATION.

Sect. 339. Art. 1. THREE cylindric wooden Veffels were funk more than half their Depth into the Ground: two of them, each, 5 Feet Diameter, and 5 Feet high: the third, 8 Feet in Diameter, and 8 Feet high.

Procefs of Inflation on the Day of Afcent, viz. on Thurfday the 8th Sept, 1785.

An oblong Hole, 4 Inches by 3, was made in each Veffel: and each Hole was furnifhed with a folid wooden Plug (made tapering) 6 Inches in Length: throu' thefe the Vitriol was poured.

Befides which, there was an oblong Opening in each Veffel, large enough to admit a Workman, to diftribute the Iron equally over the Bottom, and to pour in Buckets of Water: which

Openings were well stopped, as soon as the Iron and Water were poured in.

As the vitriolic Acid is *corrosive*, burning the Skin or Cloaths; the following Precautions were taken.

An occasional moveable Tub was provided, 3 Feet high, and 3 wide: in the Center of whose Bottom was an oblong Aperture, equal to that in each of the Vessels: a corresponding Tin Tube, 6 Inches long, and narrowing to the Bottom, was nailed by its Border on the Inside of the occasional Tub; so as to go easily into any of the oblong Holes.

A Bottle of Vitriol being brought in its Basket by two Men, and made to rest on the Top of one of the fermenting Vessels; a third Assistant held the occasional Tub in his Hands, with the Plug-Staff fastened in the Aperture of the Tin Tube; and the Instant a fourth Person opened the Hole in the fermenting Vessel; the Assistant placed the Tin Tube in the Hole, keeping the Plug tight, to prevent the Escape of Gas.

The Bottle of Vitriol was then immediately poured into the occasional Tub: and the Bottle being removed, the Plug-Staff was taken out, and the Vitriol suffered to run into the fermenting Vessel: the Assistant watching for the Instant when the Vitriol was run out, in order to *force in* the Plug-Staff again, and prevent the Escape of Gas: after which, the Tub was rinced with a few Quarts of Water, let also into the Vessel.

The same Tub was then removed: the oblong Hole in the fermenting Vessel instantly covered; and, by driving down the solid wooden Plug,

continued

continued *Air-tight*; by Means of moist Clay, and a little Water, kept purposely on the Tops of each Vessel, to discover by the Bubbles, whether Gass escaped.

In these Vessels, early on the Morning of the Inflation, were distributed 20 Hundred Weight, at 120lb. Averdupoise to the Hundred, consisting of cast Iron-Filings, and of a Mixture of Cannon-Borings. 20 Hundred Weight of Iron-Turnings.

The Borings were bright and fresh when thrown into the Water: and any Bits of Wood that swam, were skimmed off.

Rusty Iron emits Gass, that is heavier than common Air, and therefore is improper.

At the same Time, 16 Bottles of concentrated vitriolic Acid, or as it is improperly called Oil of Vitriol, were brought in their Packages near the Place, to be ready for Use: each Bottle at an Average containing 112 Pounds Averdupoise, of Vitriol: each full Bottle and Package together weighing from 136 to 148 Pounds. 16 Bottles of Vitriol.

339. 2. To the Iron in each Vessel, was then poured a Quantity of Water, which was measured in the Proportion of about 4 to 1: i. e. 4 *Pints* of Water to one *Pound*, of the vitriolic Acid. 4 Pints of Water to a Pound Averdupoise of Acid.

The Height of Water and Iron in each Vessel, being then gaged, was about 14 Inches.

In a Line with the two smaller Vessels, and between them, was fixed another wooden Vessel or Cistern, filled with Water.

(N. B. Fresh Water ought to have flowed continually into it, and to have run over the Top of the Cistern: for the same Quantity being once saturated, Improvements suggested.

faturated, can no longer abforb the alcaline and fixed Air to be feparated from the Gafs before the latter enters the Balloon.)

In the Ciftern was fixed a Stage, confifting of 4 long Feet, (reaching to the Bottom of the Ciftern,) nailed at their upper Ends to the Infide of an inverted Tub or Funnel, fo placed over the Center of the Ciftern, that 3 Inches of the lower Part of the Rim of the Funnel were under the Surface of the Ciftern-Water: the Funnel was *cylindric*, 3 Feet acrofs, and 2 Feet high.

An Open was cut, 1 Foot Diameter, in the Bottom of the inverted Funnel: on the Circumference of which was nailed a Tin-Cylinder or common Conductor, 2 Feet high: and at a *certain* Angle, as moft convenient, was foldered a cylindric Arm, of equal Diameter, and 1 Foot long; having a Lip, Ring or Rim, on its outward circular Edge.

Round this Rim was faftened a varnifhed Linen Tube, of equal Diameter with the Cylinder.

At a fmall Diftance, about a Yard from the Ciftern, ftood a flender Stillage, 3 Feet high; on which was fupported a detached Tin-Cylinder or Connecter, 1 Foot long and 1 Foot Diameter, made with a Rim at each End: in the Center of whofe lower Side was foldered, at right Angles, another Tin-Cylinder or Evacuatory, 6 Inches long and 6 wide: its Ufe is to let out any Water, that the Heat of the Mixture might caufe to boil and rife up out of the fermenting Veffels: and thus be *evacuated*, without entering the Balloon: or, if condenfed in the Balloon, might run out by the fame Orifice.

340. The

The oppofite End of the varnifhed Linen Tube was faftened round one End of the detached Cylinder on the Stillage: and round the other, was tyed the Neck or Bottom-Opening of the Balloon.

Each of the 2 fmaller fermenting Veffels was furnifhed with a cylindric Tin-Tube; each Tube 4 Inches and a half Diameter, nailed on the Outfide of a circular Opening in the Top or Head of each Veffel; communicating by additional rectangular Bends under the Funnel and Water in the Ciftern: the great fermenting Veffel had 2 Tubes, each 4 Feet and a half Diameter; communicating with the Funnel.

340. The Procefs woud have been more complete, if the fermenting Veffels had been funk till their Tops were even with the Ground: and plaiftered round their Outfides with foft moift Clay, fix Inches thick, to keep them Air-tight.

Alfo, if the common Conductor had been only 1 Foot high: its horizontal or rectangular Arm only 6 Inches long: the Linen Trunk but 3 Feet, joining the Connecter on the Stillage 1 Foot high, to communicate with the Neck of the Balloon; which Neck fhoud be 3 Yards in Length, and its circular Opening 1 Foot, at leaft in Diameter.

CHAPTER

CHAPTER LXVIII.

Inflation began about X. in the Morning.

Section 341. THE Process of inflating the Balloon began about X. in the Morning, by pouring 4 Bottles of Vitriol, immediately one after the other, into the occasional Tub, properly placed over one of the smaller fermenting Vessels: the Tub being instantly rinced with a few Quarts of Water, which was suffered to fall into the same Vessel.

The oblong Hole was left purposely open for a Minute, till the strong Smell of the Gass was perceived above the Orifice: i. e. till the Gass had pressed out all the common Air that remained floating over the Surface of the Mixture in the fermenting Vessel: which Smell being *plainly perceived*, the *solid* Plug was immediately *driven* down.

And presently the Gass was known to press forward with an elastic Force throu' the Tin Conductor, by the Motion it communicated to the Surface of the Water in the Cistern: thence upwards throu' the common Conductor: at its Departure from both of which throu' the Linen Trunk, and Neck into the Balloon, the Gass makes a guggling obtuse Sound by quick Intervals according to the Quantity of Gass protruded.

And as the Intervals encreased, a Judgment was formed, that the Operation began to be less vigorous: and consequently that it became necessary, either to renew it by an Addition of more Vitriol and Water in the same Vessel, or to set the other small Vessel in Fermentation, the latter

ter of which Mr. Lunardi preferred: this happened about half an Hour after the Vitriol was poured into the firſt Veſſel.

342. After the ſecond half Hour, eight Bottles were poured, by four at a Time, into the great Veſſel.

And at one o'Clock, the Balloon, without any farther Trouble was beautifully inflated.

No Iron Rods were uſed to ſtir up the Borings or Filings at the Bottom of the Veſſels: the Vitriol being found ſo heavy as to penetrate them as faſt as the Iron, contiguous to the Vitriol, had parted with its Gaſs.

At each of the two former Inflations, a ſimilar Accident happened which may be imputed to the ſame Cauſe.

343. During the firſt Inflation, the ſolid oblong wooden Plug fell into one of the fermenting Veſſels: the hot Vapour, forcibly iſſuing from the Orifice, was condenſed in the Form of a *white* Smoke; which being miſtaken by the Company, a Cry was immediately heard of Fire, Fire: on which the Workmen retreated. Mr. Lunardi incautiouſly thruſt his Arm into the Orifice to extract the Plug: at the ſame Time being much burnt, and failing in the Attempt; the Gaſs continued to eſcape, till a new Plug was prepared.

344. During the ſecond Inflation, one of the Plugs being driven too forcibly; it was with Difficulty extricated, by the Strokes of a Hammer againſt the Sides of it, which tended at the ſame Time to diſplace the Boards forming the Top or Head of the Veſſel: and, a little afterwards, occaſioned it to burſt, unexpectedly

edly INWARDS, (*a*) rendering the Veſſel uſeleſs for the Purpoſe of Inflation.

Obſervation. Therefore inſtead of the ſolid oblong wooden Plug, a circular Hole, 4 Inches Diameter ſhoud be drilled in each Veſſel: and a correſponding ſolid wooden Plug 8 Inches long, 5 Diameter at the upper Part, and tapering to near 3 at the Bottom, ſhoud be prepared by the Turner.

In the upper Part of the Solid ſhoud be turned an inſide Screw, to which an outſide Screw of the circular Plug-Staff, made of Oak, Aſh, or other heavy Wood, 4 Feet long, and 4 Inches Diameter, ſhoud be adapted: the Worm of the Screw to be 5 Inches long.

A wooden Peg of Aſh, about a Quarter of an Inch Diameter, may be put throu' a Hole near the Top of the Staff, as a Handle.

A Lever of ſuch a Length and Weight will probably anſwer every Intention, as no ſudden Blows will be required to *faſten or extract it*.

The occaſional Tub, Tube, Plug, and Staff, ſhoud be faſhioned after this Model.

345 *The Price of the Iron and Vitriol for Inflation.*

	£	s	d
2000lb. of Iron Filings or Borings (*b*) delivered on the Spot, at 6s. a Hundred,	6	0	0
16 Bottles of Vitriol, at an Average 38s. a Bottle	30	8	0
Concomitant Expences,	3	12	0
£. Total	40	0	0

Obſervation

(*a*) This was owing to the cool Air ruſhing in to ſupply the Tendency to a Vacuum by the Expanſion of hot Steam, with the extricated Gaſs.

The Accident proves that no Danger is to be dreaded from EXPANSION of the Gaſs.

(*b*) From *Berſham-Forge* near *Wrexham*, where there is always a ſufficient Quantity.

Obſervation 1. A great Saving might be made by conducting the Proceſs in a different Manner.

The Author making two Journies to Mancheſter, purpoſely to obſerve the Proceſs by Mr. Sadler; found that his Balloon was inflated in two Hours each Time; by Means only of the two ſmaller *identical* fermenting Veſſels which Mr. Lunardi afterwards purchaſed: but the Levity procured by the former, tho' he alſo expended 16 Bottles, was by no Means ſo great as that gained with the Aſſiſtance of the great Veſſel.

It has likewiſe been remarked by the Author, who has made ſeveral Experiments to this End, that the Veſſels always continued in Fermentation and Ebullition, with a *quick Pulſation*, for at leaſt 24, and commonly during 48 Hours, after the Inflation was completed.

And, that not more than the Depth of *half an Inch* of Filings had been *calcined* during the Operation: the reſt being perfectly *bright*, and untouched by the Acid.

Obſervation. 2. If therefore one Inch in Depth of Filings, be ſpread over the Bottom of each of the *ſmaller* Veſſels only; the proper Quantity of Water poured in; and *not more* than two Bottles of Acid uſed at once, in each Veſſel; alſo, as ſoon as the Fermentation begins to decline; other two Bottles, and a proportionable Supply of Water be added; if ſuffered to work double, triple, or quadruple the Time;—the Inflation will be as great, if not greater, for Inſtance, in ſix Hours with eight Bottles, and two ſmall *Tubs*, as it woud in three Hours, with 16 Bottles, in the *ſame Veſſels*.

The small conducting Tin Tubes ought instead of four and a half, to be nine Inches Diameter: by which Means there will be no violent Pressure of Gafs to endanger the Bursting of the Vessels: particularly if the Gafs is not suffered to descend; but, on the contrary, according to Instructions already given, either to rise, or move, in an horizontal Direction, past the Evacuatory, into the Balloon.

346. The Workmen may begin the Operation at twelve at Night, or at six in the Morning: and the Time previously fixed for the Exhibition, may be eight or ten Hours after the Operation has commenced.

The Necessity of a Current of fresh Water, throu' a Pipe of at least half Inch Bore, the larger the better, to supply the overflowing Cistern, cannot be too much *insisted* on: as the Levity of the Gafs almost wholly depends upon so trivial a Circumstance, as that of having a plentiful Supply of *cold fresh* and *soft* Water.

347. *Observation* 3. Supposing the Balloon AIR-TIGHT, near half the Expence is thus saved in the Inflation.

Besides the greater Probability of CALM Weather for the Inflation, if completed before X. in the Morning, more Time is given to remedy Accidents, and rectify Mistakes: the Warmth of the Air likewise encreases.

But above all; if an upper Current carry the Balloon to Sea, the Aironaut may, (as before mentioned) drop into the Sea-Breeze, which will waft him safe back till IV. in the Afternoon, or even later.

CHAPTER

CHAPTER LXIX.

MENSURATION OF HEIGHTS.

Section 348. **R**ULES for calculating the Height of Mountains, when applied to those elevated Stations in the Atmosphere *attainable* only by Means of the Balloon, will henceforward become more useful, and be more frequently practised: as the Lives of Aironauts *may* depend on a Knowledge of their *Height* above the Earth; which, not being determinable by *Sight*, in *all Weathers*, or at all Times, must be referred to the *Barometer* and *Thermometers*, they carry up with them.

Rules for calculating Heights by Means of the Barometer and Thermometers.

De Luc, Horseley, Maskelyne, Shuckburgh, and Roy, have each written ABLY on the Subject, in the *Transactions:* tho' few have either Leisure or Inclination to follow them.

Sir George Shuckburgh has made successful Attempts to smooth the Way, by Examples and Tables, yet is still too concise for actual Learners, and the Generality of those who will have Spirit enough to go before the Calculators in exploring the Atmosphere; but cannot dedicate sufficient Leisure to overtake them in their Studies.

Each may therefore assist the other.

349. Whoever is at the Trouble of comparing the Observations made by Shuckburgh, with the Directions here given, will find that the latter contains the *Essentials* of the former, with this material Difference, that the Investigation moves

here

here by Steps, which are all pointed out to the Learner; and not by Strides.

Each Step is felf evident: and, by carrying Conviction to the Mind, is juſt what the Mind itſelf woud make uſe of, in the Attainment of any *diſtant* Truth.

To do every Juſtice to Sir George, the Merit of whoſe Performance wants no Eulogium; his three Precepts are copied; tho' rather as a Memorandum for thoſe who underſtand the Methods; than as plain Directions for ſuch as are yet to learn them.

It will be found likewiſe, that the firſt, ſecond, and third Tables are greatly enlarged: being calculated for thoſe *extreme* Temperatures, and Heights, which the Balloon *only* can attempt to reach: and the third Table, for greater Diſpatch in computing the Expanſion of the Air.

The Foundation and Conſtruction of each Table, is alſo methodically traced and elucidated.

CHAPTER LXX.

METHODS TO ASCERTAIN THE TRUE HEIGHT.

Section 350. METHODS to be purſued on taking and comparing Heights, in order to aſcertain the true Height of any Station in the Atmoſphere, by the Barometer and Thermometers.

For this Purpoſe it is neceſſary, 1ſt, to provide

vide a Barometer, (whose Bulb or Cistern is *large* enough to contain all the Quicksilver in the Tube;)—into the Frame of which, a Thermometer, on *Farenheit's* Scale, is to be fixed or *attached*.

The Use of the *attached Thermometer* is to point out the Temperature of the Barometer.

2d. A second or *detached Thermometer* is also to be provided.(*a*)

This is to be hung in the Shade at the Distance of a Yard (or two) from the other:—to shew the *general* Temperature of the Air at the same Time and Place: and may be called the *Air Thermometer*.

A proper Person, on the Ground, having a good Watch, with Pen Ink and Paper at Hand, is to attend the Instruments *below* every ten Minutes, (or at any other *preconcerted* Intervals of Time,) putting down,

1st. The Time of each Observation.

2d. The Point at which the Quicksilver stands in the Barometer.

3d. The Degree of Temperature of the *attached* Thermometer.

4th, and lastly, the Degree of Temperature of the *detached* or *Air-*Thermometer.

This Employment is to be carefully attended to; during the Time, that *similar* Observations, by *preconcerted* Agreement, are making, with three other *similar* Instruments, on the Top of the Mountain, or any elevated Station in the Atmosphere,

(*a*) The *detached* Thermometer might be protected from the *Sun*, by being swung a few Inches *below* the Car of the Balloon by means of an *Opening* made purposely throu' the Center of the Car.

sphere, by Means of the *Balloon*; and to be written with a *red Lead* Pencil, in a Patent Asses Skin Pocket Book.

The Instruments to be compared on Return from the Mountain, or upper Station.

Each single Observation, made with one Set of Instruments *below*, is to be compared with each single corresponding Observation, made with the other Set *above*.

And two Observations are said to *correspond*, when both are made *nearly* at the *same* Time, the one *below*, and the other *above*.

351. Take Shuckburgh's first Example, (Ph. Tr. for 1777, 2d Part, Page 577.) viz.

"Let the Point at which the Quicksilver stands in the Barometer, on the Ground, be 29 Inches 4 tenths: the attached Thermometer 50 Degrees of Temperature, and the Air Thermometer, or general Temperature of the Air 45°: at the same Time, that at the Top of the Mountain, or other elevated Station in the Atmosphere, the Barometer stands at 25 Inches 19 Tenths, the attached Thermometer at 46°, and the Air Thermometer at 39° and $\frac{1}{2}$: required the upper Height in English Feet."

Rules for the Work: and Practice of the first Example.

352. The Work is divided into three Stages. The End proposed in this first Stage is to bring the colder Barometer, to the same *Expansion* or *Temperature* with the *other*.

353. 1st. Step. First, write down the Observation made on the Ground, or at the Bottom of the Mountain, thus:

BELOW. Barometer, 29 Inches 4 Tenths. attached Thermometer, 50 Degrees. Air Thermometer, 45°.

354. 2d. Step. Secondly, write down the Observation

fervation made at the Top of the Mountain, or upper Station in the Atmosphere, thus:

ABOVE. Barometer, 25 Inches, .19 Tenths, attached Thermometer, 46°. Air Thermometer, 29 ½.

355. 3d Step. Subtract the *colder attached* Thermometer, from the other attached Thermometer, thus: 46 colder from 50 warmer, and there remains 4° warmer, viz. the Number of Degrees of Temperature to which the *colder* Barometer must be *expanded*, before it becomes equal in Temperature to the *warmer* Barometer: each Barometer being always supposed *equal* in Temperature with its *attached* Thermometer.

356. 4th Step. Give the *colder* Barometer the same *Temperature* with the warmer: or, which amounts to the same, give the *colder* Barometer that *Expansion* which is communicated by the Addition of 4 Degrees of Temperature.

Both Barometers will then have the same *Temperature*, or *Expansion*, viz. an Expansion equal to the warmer Barometer.

This is to be done by referring to the first Table, for the Application of which there are separate Instructions: see the Explanation of the first Table. *(a)*

O o   CHAPTER

(a) Foundation of the first Table.

(Ph. Tr. for 1777, Part 2d, Page 567.)—It was found by Experiment that the Decimal — — .000262 was the Expansion *on* 30 Inches of Quicksilver, *with* each Degree of Temperature from freezing to boiling Water: also, the Decimal — — .000042 was the Expansion *on* 30 Inches of the Glass Tube (containing the Quicksilver), *with* each Degree of Temperature: therefore by Addition, — .000304 or by taking only 4 Decimals, — — .0003

is

CHAPTER LXXI.

USE AND PRACTICE OF THE FIRST TABLE, IN THE FIRST EXAMPLE.

The USE.

Section 357. TO find the Expansion of Quick-silver, and of the barometric Tube in which it is contained: or, in other Words, to find the Point to which the Quick-silver will rise in the Tube, (in Parts of an Inch) with a given additional Temperature, on Farenheit's Scale.

The Question in the first Example is, (Ph. Tr. for 1777, Page 578;)

To find the Expansion that arises, *with* the Addition of 4 Degrees of Heat, *on* the *colder* Barometer resting at Inches 25 .19 Tenths, in order to give it an Expansion equal to that of another Barometer, 4 Degrees warmer than the former: the Temperature of *each* Barometer, being indicated by its respective *attached* Thermometer.

N.B. During the Application of the first Table, the Investigation moves forward two Steps only, viz. the 4th and 5th.

The 4th Step, applied in the first Example.

358. The *Order* to be observed in finding the Expansion is the Expansion *on* 30 Inches of Quicksilver, and the Glass Tube containing it, *with* each Degree of Temperature.

Construction of the first Table.

Thus any vertical Number, shewing the Expansion, may be readily *formed*, by *doubling*, *first*, the Number immediately under each Inch for the Expansion below it: and *afterwards*, by adding the Number immediately under each Inch, to the Expansion last found.

Note: The vertical Columns, below each Inch of Quicksilver shew the Expansion *on* that Inch, *with* corresponding Degrees

PRACTICE OF THE FIRST TABLE.

Expanſion of the Quickſilver, with 4 Degrees on Inches 25 .19 Tenths of the Barometer.

1ſt. Find the Expanſion, With 4° on 25 Inches only.

Then in order to obtain with 4° on .19, begin

2d. With 4° on 1 Inch above 25 Inches, i. e. on the 26th Inch.

3d. With 4° on .1, i. e. one Tenth of an Inch above 25 Inches: and laſtly,

4th. With 4° on .19, Tenths above 25 Inches.

The PRACTICE.

359. 1ſt. In the *firſt* Table, *with* 4 Degrees on the left Hand vertical Column, and with 25 Inches, along the upper Range; at the Point of Meeting, is the Anſwer .0101 (*a*) viz. the Expanſion, or Riſe of the Quickſilver ſtanding at 25 Inches, and receiving an additional Heat of 4°: the Anſwer .0101 being the Expreſſion for the ten thouſand one hundredth Part of an Inch, (viz. in Height, by Expanſion.)

360. Add this Number, .0101, Part of an Inch, or Riſe by Expanſion, to the Barometer reſting at Inches 25, .19 Tenths, Units under Units, &c. thus: .0101.

361. 2d. Now, in order to obtain the Expanſion *with* 4 Degrees, *on* .19 Tenths i. e. the nine hundred and tenth Part of an Inch of Quickſilver in the Tube (above 25 Inches,) it muſt be conſidered, where it ought to be found in the firſt Table.

Tenths

Degrees of Temperature indicated by the Thermometer in the Column to the left Hand. Example: to find the Expanſion *on* 30 Inches of Quickſilver *with* 1 Degree of Temperature: the Anſwer in the Table is .003: i. e. ſuch Expanſion raiſes the Quickſilver the 3000th Part of an Inch.

(*a*) There is ſeldom Occaſion to take more than the three firſt Decimals out of the Table, the Remainder being of *little value.*

PRACTICE OF THE FIRST TABLE,

Tenths of 1 Inch, above 25 Inches, it must be observed, are at some intermediate Point between 25 and 26 Inches; that is, above 25, yet not so high as 26, or more than 25, yet less than 26.

Therefore, to find the Expansion *with* 4 Degrees, *on* 1 Inch above 25, i. e. on the 26th Inch; look in the Table, first, *with* 4 Degrees on 25 Inches: then *with* 4 Degrees on 26 Inches. The respective Numbers are .0101 and .0105.

And by taking the Expansion *with* 4° on 25 Inches, from the Expansion, *with* 4° *on* 26 Inches, thus;

Expansion $\begin{cases} .0101 \text{ on 25 Inches,} \\ .0105 \text{ on 26 Inches,} \end{cases}$

The Remainder .0004 is the Expansion with 4° on 1 Inch, above 25, i. e. on the 26th Inch.

362. 3d. To find the Expansion, with 4° on .1 above 25 Inches; add a Cypher and decimal Point to the former Answer, which then becomes .00004, viz. the Expansion, with 4° on one Tenth, above 25 Inches.

363. 4th. Lastly, to obtain the Expansion *with* 4°, *on* .19, above 25 Inches, say: If one Tenth of an Inch, above 25 Inches, gives this Expansion viz. 00004, what Expansion will nineteen Tenths above 25, give? answer .19 Tenths more; thus:
If .1   :   .00004 :: .19?
                .19
            ———————
              00036
              0004
            ———————
        .00076; then, in order to have
        (See Page 288)

THE FIRST TABLE:
SHEWING THE EXPANSION WITH HEAT ON INCHES OF THE BAROMETER.

	9	10	11	12	13	14	15	16
1	.00091	.00102	.00112	.00122	.00132	.00142	.00152	.00162
2	.00182	.00204	.00224	.00244	.00264	.00284	.00304	.00324
3	.00273	.00306	.00336	.00366	.00396	.00426	.00456	.00486
4	.00364	.00408	.00448	.00488	.00528	.00568	.00608	.00648
5	.00455	.00510	.00560	.00610	.00660	.00710	.00760	.00810
6	.00546	.00612	.00672	.00732	.00792	.00852	.00912	.00972
7	.00637	.00714	.00784	.00854	.00924	.00994	.01064	.01134
8	.00728	.00816	.00896	.00976	.01056	.01136	.01216	.01296
9	.00819	.00918	.01008	.01098	.01188	.01278	.01368	.01458
10	.00910	.01020	.01120	.01220	.01320	.01420	.01520	.01620
11	.01001	.01122	.01232	.01342	.01452	.01562	.01672	.01782
12	.01092	.01224	.01344	.01464	.01584	.01704	.01824	.01944
13	.01183	.01326	.01456	.01586	.01716	.01846	.01976	.02106
14	.01274	.01428	.01568	.01708	.01848	.01988	.02128	.02268
15	.01365	.01530	.01680	.01830	.01980	.02130	.02280	.02430
16	.01456	.01632	.01792	.01952	.02112	.02272	.02432	.02592
17	.01547	.01734	.01904	.02074	.02244	.02414	.02584	.02754
18	.01638	.01836	.02016	.02196	.02376	.02556	.02736	.02916
19	.01729	.01938	.02128	.02318	.02508	.02698	.02888	.03078
20	.01820	.02040	.02240	.02440	.02640	.02840	.03040	.03240
21	.01911	.02142	.02352	.02562	.02772	.02982	.03192	.03402
22	.02002	.02244	.02464	.02684	.02904	.03124	.03344	.03564
23	.02093	.02346	.02576	.02806	.03036	.03266	.03496	.03726
24	.02184	.02448	.02688	.02928	.03168	.03408	.03648	.03888
25	.02275	.02550	.02800	.03050	.03300	.03550	.03800	.04050
26	.02366	.02652	.02912	.03172	.03432	.03692	.03952	.04212
27	.02457	.02754	.03024	.03294	.03564	.03834	.04104	.04374
28	.02548	.02856	.03136	.03416	.03696	.03976	.04256	.04536
29	.02639	.02958	.03248	.03538	.03828	.04118	.04408	.04698
30	.02730	.03060	.03360	.03660	.03960	.04260	.04560	.04860
31	.02821	.03162	.03472	.03782	.04092	.04402	.04712	.05022
32	.02912	.03264	.03584	.03904	.04224	.04544	.04864	.05184
33	.03003	.03366	.03696	.04026	.04356	.04686	.05016	.05346
34	.03094	.03468	.03808	.04148	.04488	.04828	.05168	.05508
35	.03185	.03570	.03920	.04270	.04620	.04970	.05320	.05670
36	.03276	.03672	.04032	.04392	.04752	.05112	.05472	.05832
37	.03367	.03774	.04144	.04514	.04884	.05254	.05624	.05994
38	.03458	.03876	.04256	.04636	.05016	.05396	.05776	.06156
39	.03549	.03978	.04368	.04758	.05148	.05538	.05928	.06318
40	.03640	.04080	.04480	.04880	.05280	.05680	.06080	.06480

DEGREES OF THE THERMOMETER, FROM 1 TO 40, ON FARENHEIT'S SCALE.

THE FIRST TABLE CONTINUED:
SHEWING THE EXPANSION WITH HEAT ON INCHES OF THE BAROMETER.

DEGREES OF THE THERMOMETER, FROM 1 TO 40, ON FARENHEIT'S SCALE.	17	18	19	20	21	22	23	24
1	.00172	.00182	.00192	.00203	.00213	.00223	.00233	.00243
2	.00344	.00364	.00384	.00406	.00426	.00446	.00466	.00486
3	.00516	.00546	.00576	.00609	.00639	.00669	.00699	.00729
4	.00688	.00728	.00768	.00812	.00852	.00892	.00932	.00972
5	.00860	.00910	.00960	.01015	.01065	.01115	.01165	.01215
6	.01032	.01092	.01152	.01218	.01278	.01338	.01398	.01458
7	.01204	.01274	.01344	.01421	.01491	.01561	.01631	.01701
8	.01376	.01456	.01536	.01624	.01704	.01784	.01864	.01944
9	.01548	.01638	.01728	.01827	.01917	.02007	.02097	.02187
10	.01720	.01820	.01920	.02030	.02130	.02230	.02330	.02430
11	.01892	.02002	.02112	.02233	.02343	.02453	.02563	.02673
12	.02064	.02184	.02304	.02436	.02556	.02676	.02796	.02916
13	.02236	.02366	.02496	.02639	.02769	.02899	.03029	.03159
14	.02408	.02548	.02688	.02842	.02982	.03122	.03262	.03402
15	.02580	.02730	.02880	.03045	.03195	.03345	.03495	.03645
16	.02752	.02912	.03072	.03248	.03408	.03568	.03728	.03888
17	.02924	.03094	.03264	.03451	.03621	.03791	.03961	.04131
18	.03096	.03276	.03456	.03654	.03834	.04014	.04194	.04374
19	.03268	.03458	.03648	.03857	.04047	.04237	.04427	.04617
20	.03440	.03640	.03840	.04060	.04260	.04460	.04660	.04860
21	.03612	.03822	.04032	.04263	.04473	.04683	.04893	.05103
22	.03784	.04004	.04224	.04466	.04686	.04906	.05126	.05346
23	.03956	.04186	.04416	.04669	.04899	.05129	.05359	.05589
24	.04128	.04368	.04608	.04872	.05112	.05352	.05592	.05832
25	.04300	.04550	.04800	.05075	.05325	.05575	.05825	.06075
26	.04472	.04732	.04992	.05278	.05538	.05798	.06058	.06318
27	.04644	.04914	.05184	.05481	.05751	.06021	.06291	.06561
28	.04816	.05096	.05376	.05684	.05964	.06244	.06524	.06804
29	.04988	.05278	.05568	.05887	.06177	.06467	.06757	.07047
30	.05160	.05460	.05760	.06090	.06390	.06690	.06990	.07290
31	.05332	.05642	.05952	.06293	.06603	.06913	.07223	.07533
32	.05504	.05824	.06144	.06496	.06816	.07139	.07456	.07776
33	.05676	.06006	.06336	.06699	.07029	.07359	.07689	.08019
34	.05848	.06188	.06528	.06902	.07242	.07582	.07922	.08262
35	.06020	.06350	.06720	.07105	.07455	.07805	.08155	.08505
36	.06192	.06534	.06912	.07308	.07668	.08028	.08388	.08748
37	.06364	.06716	.07104	.07511	.07881	.08251	.08621	.08991
38	.06536	.06892	.07296	.07714	.08094	.08474	.08854	.09234
39	.06708	.07078	.07488	.07917	.08307	.08697	.09087	.09477
40	.06880	.07260	.07680	.08120	.08520	.08920	.09320	.09720

THE FIRST TABLE CONCLUDED:
SHEWING THE EXPANSION WITH HEAT ON INCHES OF THE BAROMETER.

DEGREES OF THE THERMOMETER, FROM 1 TO 40, ON FARENHEIT'S SCALE.

	25	26	27	28	29	30	31	32
1	.00253	.00263	.00274	.00284	.00294	.00304	.00314	.00324
2	.00506	.00526	.00548	.00568	.00588	.00608	.00628	.00648
3	.00759	.00789	.00822	.00852	.00882	.00912	.00942	.00972
4	.01012	.01052	.01096	.01136	.01176	.01216	.01256	.01296
5	.01265	.01315	.01370	.01420	.01470	.01520	.01570	.01620
6	.01518	.01578	.01644	.01704	.01764	.01824	.01884	.01944
7	.01771	.01841	.01918	.01988	.02058	.02128	.02198	.02268
8	.02024	.02104	.02192	.02272	.02352	.02432	.02512	.0259
9	.02277	.02367	.02466	.02556	.02646	.02736	.02826	.02916
10	.02530	.02630	.02740	.02840	.02940	.03040	.03140	.03240
11	.02783	.02893	.03014	.03124	.03234	.03344	.03454	.03564
12	.03036	.03156	.03288	.03408	.03528	.03648	.03768	.03888
13	.03289	.03419	.03562	.03692	.03822	.03952	.04082	.04212
14	.03542	.03682	.03836	.03976	.04116	.04256	.04396	.04536
15	.03795	.03945	.04110	.04260	.04410	.04560	.04710	.04860
16	.04048	.04208	.04384	.04544	.04704	.04864	.05024	.05184
17	.04301	.04471	.04658	.04828	.04998	.05168	.05338	.05508
18	.04554	.04734	.04932	.05112	.05292	.05472	.05652	.05832
19	.04807	.04997	.05206	.05396	.05586	.05776	.05966	.06156
20	.05060	.05260	.05480	.05680	.05880	.06080	.06280	.06480
21	.05313	.05523	.05754	.05964	.06174	.06384	.06594	.06804
22	.05566	.05786	.06028	.06248	.06468	.06688	.06908	.07128
23	.05819	.06049	.06302	.06532	.06762	.06992	.07222	.07452
24	.06072	.06312	.06576	.06816	.07056	.07296	.07536	.07776
25	.06325	.06575	.06850	.07100	.07350	.07600	.07850	.08100
26	.06578	.06838	.07124	.07384	.07644	.07904	.08164	.08424
27	.06831	.07101	.07398	.07668	.07938	.08208	.08478	.08748
28	.07084	.07364	.07672	.07952	.08232	.08512	.08792	.09072
29	.07337	.07627	.07946	.08236	.08526	.08816	.09106	.09396
30	.07590	.07890	.08220	.08520	.08820	.09120	.09420	.09720
31	.07843	.08153	.08494	.08804	.09114	.09424	.09734	.10044
32	.08096	.08416	.08768	.09088	.09408	.09728	.10048	.10368
33	.08349	.08679	.09042	.09372	.09702	.10032	.10362	.10692
34	.08602	.08942	.09316	.09656	.09996	.10336	.10676	.11016
35	.08855	.09205	.09590	.09940	.10290	.10640	.10990	.11340
36	.09108	.09468	.09864	.10224	.10584	.10944	.11314	.11664
37	.09361	.09731	.10138	.10508	.10878	.11248	.11618	.11988
38	.09614	.09994	.10412	.10792	.11172	.11552	.11932	.12312
39	.09867	.10257	.10686	.11076	.11466	.11866	.12246	.12636
40	.10120	.10520	.10960	.11360	.11760	.12160	.12560	.12960

as many decimal Places in the Product as are contained both in the Multiplicand and Multiplier, add a Cypher and Point to the left, and the Product becomes .0000076

viz. the Expansion with 4° on 19. above 25 Inches.

The 5th Step, applied in the first Example.

364. Add this, to the former Expansion, thus:

Inches 25.19 Tenths
with 4° on .25   .0101 Expansion
with 4° on .19   .0000076 Expansion
_____

The Answer is 25.2|001076, viz. the Point at which the Quickfilver woud ftand, in the coldeft Barometer, when equally *expanded*, i. e. of the fame Temperature with the warmer. Reject all but the firft Decimal as too minute: this is feen by a Line drawn between the firft and fecond Decimal.

Practice will fhew how far to proceed, without computing the decimal Parts of an Inch, to more than 4 Places; but it is always more exact, to follow minutely the above Rules.

_____

CHAPTER LXXII.

Section 365. HAVING therefore underftood the Foundation, Conftruction, and Ufe of the firft Table; in the prefent Cafe, having alfo added the decimal Parts of an Inch juft found, for the Expanfion,—to the Inches and
Tenths,

Tenths, expressing the colder Barometer; which will then have the *same Expansion,* or *Temperature* with the warmer, thus;
Inches.
  25.19   *colder* Barometer:
   .0101 Expansion *on* the same, in Parts of an Inch with 4° of Temperature, (rejecting all but the first Decimal as too minute,)
  25.2|001 added; this Sum will express the Point at which the Quicksilver in the colder Barometer woud stand, when equally expanded, i. e. in the same Temperature, with the warmer.

366. 6th Step. Place both Barometers, now of *equal* Temperature with the warmer, together, first, the *upper* Barometer; and under it the *lower*, thus: Inches 25. 2 Tenths.
                  29. 4

END OF THE FIRST STAGE.

---

367. The Ends proposed in the *second Stage* of the Work, (the colder Barometer being *now* brought to the same Expansion or Temperature with the warmer,) are two: First, to find, (by the Application of the second Table) the Heights, in Feet and Tenths, in the Atmosphere, corresponding to the Points at which the Quicksilver stands in both Barometers, which have now the same Temperature, viz. that of the warmer equal to 50°: on a Supposition that they were both exposed to the Temperature of 31°.24, on Farenheit's Scale, which is about the Standard or freez-

ing Point, for which sole Purpose the 2d Table is calculated.

N. B. The *Second Stage* includes two Steps only, viz. the 7th and 8th.

368. 7th Step. The Barometers being placed in one View, as before directed, thus:

Upper Barometer, Inches 25 .2 Tenths.

Lower Barometer, Inches 29 .4; find, with the Temperature of 31°.24, the corresponding Heights in the Atmosphere.

This is to be done by referring to the 2d Table, for the Application of which there are separate Instructions: See the Explanation of the second Table. (a)

CHAPTER

(a) *The Foundation of the second Table.*

This Table is calculated from Briggs's Logarithms: each Number, in the second Column, being nothing more than the Logarithm—corresponding to the Point, (in the *first* Column,) at which the Quicksilver stands in the barometric Tube,—subtracted from the Logarithm of 32 Inches multiplied by 6.

Construction of the second Table.

This Table consists of three *vertical* Columns only: tho' *here* tripled, for the greater Convenience of Inspection.

The first or left Hand Column shews, in Inches and Tenths (from ten Inches) the Gradations of the Quicksilver in the barometric Tube, beginning as low as one Inch above the Surface in the Cistern, and proceeding throu' all the intermediate Points, to the unusual Extent of 32 Inches: (a) supposing

(a) *The Barometer, (to which the Scale of Heights is applied, in the 2d Column of the 2d Table) is supposed to be sunk within the Surface of the Earth, till the Quicksilver rests at 32 Inches, as appears from the last Article in the Table, viz.* 32 *Inches,* 0.00 *Feet.* 32 *Inches is therefore the Foundation of the Table, and corresponds, according to Shuckburgh, to* 1647 *Feet, under the Surface of the Sea, at low Water).*

This Depth *then being the* imaginary Level *pointed out by the Quicksilver, at the* unusual *Extent of* 32 *Inches; each* interior *Inch and Tenth of Quicksilver will correspond to a* superior *Elevation of the Instrument, in Feet and Tenths above that Level, and will include the Mensuration of the* deepest *Mines.*

For the mean *Pressure of the Barometer, at low Water, from*

CHAPTER LXXIII.

USE AND PRACTICE OF THE SECOND TABLE IN THE FIRST EXAMPLE.

The USE.

Section 369. TO find the Heights, in Feet and Tenths, in the Atmofphere, correfponding to the Points at which

the pofing likewife that the Tube is elevated in the Atmofphere, fo that the contained Quickfilver, when expofed to the Temperature of 31°. 24 of Farenheit, refts at each Point in the Table.

The fecond vertical Column gives the different Heights in Feet and Tenths, to which the barometric Tube muft be raifed above its Level at 32 Inches, in order that the contained Quickfilver, if expofed to the Temperature of 31°.24 of Farenheit, may ftand at each Point indicated in the firft Column.

The third vertical Column, gives, likewife in Feet and Tenths, the DIFFERENCE between each two adjoining Heights in the fecond Column, correfponding to a fingle Tenth (of Quickfilver): which fingle Tenth is the Difference between each two adjoining Tenths of an Inch in the firft Column.

For Example: Suppofe the Quickfilver in the barometric Tube, in the firft Column, ftands at

Inches - 16.1 anfwering to 19570.4 ⎫ Height in Feet
And again at 16.2 anfwering to 19398.4 ⎬ in the Atmo-
⎭ fphere.

Difference of .1 in Feet: remaining = 172.0

which fixteen Inches two Tenths, is a fingle Tenth more than fixteen Inches one Tenth, and will therefore anfwer to a *lefs* Height in the Atmofphere by that fingle Tenth; confidering that the lower the Quickfilver falls in the Tube, the higher muft the Barometer itfelf be raifed in the Atmofphere, in order that the Quickfilver may reft at the lower Points of the Tube. If therefore a *lefs* Height in the Atmofphere be required which fhall anfwer to one Tenth more than 16 Inches two Tenths; fubtract the Height anfwering to 16.2 from the Height anfwering to 16.1, i.e. fubtract the *lefs* Height from the *greater*, and the Remainder gives that *lefs* Height in the third Column, anfwering to the Height of one Tenth more than 16 Inches 2 Tenths, of the Barometer.

from 132 *Obfervation*s *in Italy and England, is* 30.04 *Inches*: *the Temperature of the Barometer being at* 55°, i.e. *Temperate, and that of the Air at* 62°.

the Quickfilver ftands in both Barometers, which have *now* the *fame Temperature*, viz. that of the *warmer* Barometer, on a Suppofition that they were both expofed to the Standard-Temperature of 31°.24, on Farenheit's Scale.

The PRACTICE.

The 7th Step applied in the firft Example.

370. Look at the firft Column, in the *fecond* Table, for

25.2, and the Anfwer is 6225.0 in the fecond Column; and for

29.4, and the Anfwer is 2208.2. The Anfwers are the Heights, in Feet and Tenths, in the Atmofphere, at which the Quickfilver ftands in both Barometers, with the Temperature of 31°.24: correfponding to their refpective Points, for which *fole* Purpofe this Table is calculated.

371. 8th Step. Having placed the Barometers and their correfponding Heights in the Atmofphere, fhewn by the fecond Table, at one View: fubtract the leffer from the whole Height, and there will remain the greater Height, viz. the Height correfponding to the Barometer in the elevated Station, above the Height correfponding to the Barometer, on the Ground, (both being at the Temperature of 31°.24) thus: Feet.

Inches 25.2 correfpond to 6225.0

Inches 2?.4 correfpond to 2208.2; fubtract:

—————

and the Remainder is 4016.8 viz. a Number in Feet and Tenths correfponding to the Height of the upper above the lower Barometer, both being in the Temperature of 31°.34. (See Page 295.) 372. *Now*

THE SECOND TABLE.

The 1st Column shews the Quicksilver in the barometric Tube standing at each Inch from 1 to 10, and at each Tenth from 10 to 32 Inches.

The 2d Column shews the Height of the barometric Tube, above the *imaginary Level at 32 Inches*,—*with* the Temperature of 31.24;—in Feet and Tenths, answering to Inches and Tenths of the Barometer in the first Column.

The 3d Column shews the Height in Feet and Tenths, answering to a Tenth of an Inch on the Barometer, being the DIFFERENCE between each two adjoining Heights in the 2d Column.

Inch.	Feet.	Difference.	Inch.	Feet.	Diff.	Inch.	Feet.	Diff.
1	90309.0	18061.8	12.1	25341.8	216.3	15.1	19570.4	173.1
2	72247.2	10565.4	.2	25127.4	214.4	.2	19398.4	172.0
3	61681.8	7496.4	.3	24914.7	212.7	.3	19227.5	170.9
4	54185.4	5814.6	.4	24703.7	211.0	.4	19057.7	169.8
5	48370.8	4750.9	.5	24494.4	209.3	.5	18889.1	168.6
6	43619.9	4016.8	.6	24286.7	207.7	.6	18721.5	167.6
7	39603.1	3479.5	.7	24080.7	206.0	.7	18555.0	166.5
8	36123.6	3069.2	.8	23876.4	204.3	.8	18389.6	165.4
9	33054.4	2745.4	.9	23673.6	202.8	.9	18225.5	164.1
10.0	30309.0	259.6	13.0	23472.4	201.2	16.0	18061.8	163.7
.1	30049.4	256.4	.1	23272.7	199.7	.1	17899.4	162.4
.2	29793.0	254.3	.2	23074.5	198.2	.2	17738.1	161.3
.3	29538.7	251.8	.3	22877.9	196.6	.3	17577.7	160.4
.4	29286.9	249.3	.4	22682.7	195.2	.4	17418.4	159.3
.5	29037.6	247.0	.5	22489.0	193.7	.5	17260.0	158.4
.6	28790.6	244.7	.6	22296.6	192.4	.6	17102.5	157.5
.7	28545.9	242.4	.7	22105.6	191.0	.7	16946.0	156.5
.8	28303.5	240.2	.8	21916.2	189.4	.8	16790.4	155.6
.9	28063.3	237.9	.9	21728.1	188.1	.9	16635.8	154.6
11.0	27825.4	235.8	14.0	21541.3	186.8	17.0	16482.1	153.7
.1	27589.6	233.7	.1	21355.8	185.5	.1	16329.2	152.9
.2	27355.9	231.6	.2	21171.7	184.1	.2	16177.3	151.9
.3	27124.3	229.6	.3	20988.8	182.9	.3	16026.2	151.1
.4	26894.7	227.6	.4	20807.2	181.6	.4	15876.0	150.2
.5	26667.1	225.6	.5	20626.9	180.3	.5	15726.7	149.3
.6	26441.5	223.7	.6	20447.9	179.0	.6	15578.2	148.5
.7	26217.8	221.7	.7	20269.9	178.0	.7	15430.6	147.6
.8	25996.1	220.0	.8	20093.2	176.7	.8	15283.8	146.8
.9	25776.1	218.0	.9	19917.8	175.4	.9	15137.8	146.0
12.0	25558.1		15.0	19743.5	174.3	18.0	14992.6	145.2

MENSURATION OF HEIGHTS,

THE SECOND TABLE CONTINUED.

Inch	Feet	Diff.	Inch	Feet	Diff.	Inch	Feet	Diff
18.1	14848.2	144.3	22.1	9645.5	118.1	26.1	5310.6	99.8
.2	14704.7	143.6	.2	9527.8	117.7	.2	5210.9	99.7
.3	14561.9	142.8	.3	9410.7	117.1	.3	5111.6	99.3
.4	14419.9	142.0	.4	9294.1	116.6	.4	5012.8	98.8
.5	14278.7	141.2	.5	9178.1	116.0	.5	4914.2	98.6
.6	14138.2	140.5	.6	9062.5	115.6	.6	4816.1	98.1
.7	13998.5	139.7	.7	8947.4	115.1	.7	4718.3	97.8
.8	13859.5	139.0	.8	8832.9	114.5	.8	4620.9	97.4
.9	13721.3	138.2	.9	8718.9	114.0	.9	4523.9	97.0
19.0	13583.8	137.5	23.0	8605.3	113.6	27.0	4427.2	96.7
.1	13447.0	136.8	.1	8492.3	113.0	.1	4330.8	96.4
.2	13310.9	136.1	.2	8379.7	112.6	.2	4234.9	95.9
.3	13175.6	135.3	.3	8267.6	112.7	.3	4139.2	95.7
.4	13041.1	134.5	.4	8156.0	111.6	.4	4044.0	95.2
.5	12906.9	134.2	.5	8044.9	111.1	.5	3949.0	95.0
.6	12773.6	133.3	.6	7934.3	110.6	.6	3854.5	94.5
.7	12641.0	132.6	.7	7824.1	110.2	.7	3760.2	94.3
.8	12509.1	131.9	.8	7714.4	109.7	.8	3666.3	93.9
.9	12377.8	131.3	.9	7605.1	109.3	.9	3572.7	93.6
20.0	12247.2	130.6	24.0	7496.3	108.8	28.0	3479.5	93.2
.1	12117.2	130.0	.1	7388.0	108.3	.1	3386.6	92.9
.2	11987.9	129.3	.2	7280.1	107.9	.2	3294.0	92.6
.3	11859.2	128.7	.3	7172.6	107.5	.3	3201.8	92.2
.4	11731.2	128.0	.4	7065.6	107.0	.4	3109.9	91.9
.5	11603.8	127.4	.5	6959.0	106.6	.5	3018.3	91.6
.6	11477.0	126.8	.6	6852.9	106.1	.6	2927.0	91.3
.7	11350.8	126.2	.7	6747.2	105.7	.7	2836.1	90.9
.8	11225.2	125.6	.8	6641.9	105.3	.8	2745.4	90.7
.9	11100.2	125.0	.9	6537.0	104.9	.9	2655.1	90.3
21.0	10975.8	124.4	25.0	6432.6	104.4	29.0	2565.1	90.0
.1	10852.1	123.7	.1	6328.6	104.0	.1	2475.4	89.7
.2	10728.8	123.3	.2	6225.0	103.6	.2	2386.0	89.4
.3	10606.2	122.6	.3	6121.8	103.2	.3	2296.9	89.1
.4	10484.2	122.0	.4	6019.0	102.8	.4	2208.2	88.7
.5	10362.7	121.5	.5	5916.6	102.4	.5	2119.7	88.5
.6	10241.8	120.9	.6	5814.6	102.0	.6	2031.5	88.2
.7	10121.4	120.4	.7	5713.0	101.6	.7	1943.6	87.9
.8	10001.6	119.8	.8	5611.8	101.2	.8	1856.0	87.6
.9	9882.4	119.2	.9	5511.0	100.8	.9	1768.7	87.3
22.0	9763.6	118.8	26.0	5410.4	100.6	30.0	1681.7	87.0

THE SECOND TABLE CONCLUDED.

Inch.	Feet.	Diff.	Inch.	Feet.	Diff.	Inch.	Feet.	Diff.
30.1	1595.0	86.7	30.8	996.0	84.7	31.5	410.4	82.8
.2	1508.6	86.4	.9	911.5	84.5	.6	327.8	82.6
.3	1422.4	86.2	31.0	827.3	84.2	.7	245.4	82.4
.4	1236.6	85.8	.1	743.4	83.9	.8	163.4	82.0
.5	1251.0	85.6	.2	659.7	83.7	.9	81.6	81.8
.6	1165.7	85.3	.3	576.3	83.4	32.0	00.0	81.6
.7	1080.7	85.0	.4	493.2	83.1			

372. *Now* apply the third Table, or Table for Tenths, *if neceſſary*; including two more Steps, viz. the 9th and 10th: which, being uſeleſs, in the firſt Example, are, for the preſent, omitted.

373. An Explanation of the third Table, or Table for Tenths, is, however, for the Sake of *Order*, here ſubjoined. *(a)* (See Page 298.)

   (a) Foundation of the Table for Tenths.
 The Height, in *Feet*, correſponding to the Expanſion on the Tenth of an Inch of Quickſilver with the Temperature of 31°.24 (as in the 3d Column of the 2d Table) are reduced by this Table into a ten Times leſs Number of Feet: and the Tenth of an Inch (of Quickſilver) is alſo again divided into *ten* more Parts: in order to ſhew, in a ten Times leſs Number of *ſuch* Feet, the Expanſion correſponding to any of thoſe Parts into which the *Tenth* of an Inch (of Quickſilver) has been divided.
   Conſtruction and Uſe of the Table for Tenths.
 1. The Figures in the left vertical Column ſhew the Height in *Feet*, (from 81 to 130) correſponding to a ſingle Tenth of an Inch of Quickſilver, viz. to the higher of two adjoining Tenths, as in the 3d Column of the 2d Table.
 2. The Figures, along the upper horizontal Line, ſhew the Number of Parts into which the Tenth of an Inch has been divided.
 3. The Figures, at the Point of Meeting, expreſs, in a ten Times leſs Number, of *the Feet* in the left vertical Column, the Expanſion correſponding to any of thoſe Parts, into which the Tenth of an Inch (of Quickſilver) has been divided.
 Thus: 90 is a *Number of Feet* called 9 Tenths of 100: but the *Tenths* are *Feet*, and not Tenths of a Foot.

THE THIRD TABLE, OR TABLE FOR TENTHS:

Serving to compleat the 2d Table, on Expansion of the Barometer, with the Temperature of 31°.24.

1. The upper horizontal Figures shew the Number of Parts into which the Tenth of an Inch has been divided.
2. The Figures in the left vertical Column express the Height in FEET, (above the imaginary Level, at 32 Inches of the Barometer,) or Expansion corresponding to a single Tenth of an Inch of Quicksilver.
3. The FEET in the Place of Meeting are called TENTHS: thus, 90 Feet are 9 Tenths of 100 Feet.

Feet.	Parts into which the Tenth of an Inch is divided.								
	$\frac{1}{10}$	$\frac{2}{10}$	$\frac{3}{10}$	$\frac{4}{10}$	$\frac{5}{10}$	$\frac{6}{10}$	$\frac{7}{10}$	$\frac{8}{10}$	$\frac{9}{10}$
81	8	16	24	32	40	49	57	65	73
82	8	16	25	33	41	49	57	66	74
83	8	17	25	33	41	50	58	66	75
84	8	17	25	34	42	50	59	67	76
85	8	17	25	34	42	51	59	68	76
86	9	17	26	34	43	52	60	69	77
87	9	17	26	35	43	52	61	70	78
88	9	18	26	35	44	53	62	70	79
89	9	18	27	36	44	53	62	71	80
90	9	18	27	36	45	54	63	72	81
91	9	18	27	36	45	55	64	73	82
92	9	18	28	37	46	55	64	74	83
93	9	19	28	37	46	56	65	74	84
94	9	19	28	38	47	56	66	75	85
95	9	19	28	38	47	57	66	76	85
96	10	19	29	38	48	58	67	77	86
97	10	19	29	39	48	58	68	78	87
98	10	20	29	39	49	59	69	78	88
99	10	20	30	40	49	59	69	79	89
100	10	20	30	40	50	60	70	80	90
101	10	20	30	40	50	61	71	81	91
102	10	20	31	41	51	61	71	82	92
103	10	21	31	41	51	62	72	82	93
104	10	21	31	42	52	62	73	83	94
105	10	21	31	42	52	63	73	84	94

BY A BAROMETER AND THERMOMETERS.

THE TABLE FOR TENTHS CONCLUDED.

Feet.	Parts into which the Tenth of an Inch is divided.								
	$\frac{1}{10}$	$\frac{2}{10}$	$\frac{3}{10}$	$\frac{4}{10}$	$\frac{5}{10}$	$\frac{6}{10}$	$\frac{7}{10}$	$\frac{8}{10}$	$\frac{9}{10}$
106	11	21	32	42	53	64	74	85	95
107	11	21	32	43	53	64	75	86	96
108	11	22	32	43	54	65	76	86	97
109	11	22	33	44	54	65	76	87	98
110	11	22	33	44	55	66	77	88	99
111	11	22	33	44	55	67	78	89	100
112	11	22	34	45	56	67	78	90	101
113	11	23	34	45	56	68	79	90	102
114	11	23	34	46	57	68	80	91	103
115	11	23	34	46	57	69	80	92	103
116	12	23	35	46	58	70	81	93	104
117	12	23	35	47	58	70	82	94	105
118	12	24	35	47	59	71	83	94	106
119	12	24	36	48	59	71	83	95	107
120	12	24	36	48	60	72	84	96	108
121	12	24	36	48	60	73	85	97	109
122	12	24	37	49	61	73	85	98	110
123	12	25	37	49	61	74	86	98	111
124	12	25	37	50	62	74	87	99	112
125	12	25	37	50	62	75	87	100	112
126	13	25	38	50	63	76	88	101	113
127	13	25	38	51	63	76	89	102	114
128	13	26	38	51	64	77	90	102	115
129	13	26	39	52	64	77	90	103	116
130	13	26	39	52	65	78	91	104	117

END OF THE SECOND STAGE.

374. The Ends propofed in the third and laft Stage of the Work, are, firft, to add the *general* Temperatures of the Air, or detached Air-Thermometers, at each Place of Obfervation *above* and *below*, into one Sum.

Secondly, to divide that Sum: each Moiety of which is called the *mean Temperature* of the Air.

Thirdly, to apply that Moiety to each Barometer, (both of which have been already brought to the Standard-Temperature of 31°. 24;) in order to prove whether the Moiety (or Quantity of Heat affigned to each Barometer by the *general* Temperature of the Air) *exceeded, fell fhort of*, or equalled the Standard-Temperature of the Barometers, by the 2d Table.

And fourthly, from the Moiety or mean Temperature of the Air, to find the true Height of the upper Barometer: which Temperature refolves itfelf into three Cafes.

375. 1ft. If the Moiety or mean Temperature of of the Air is greater than the Standard Temperature, viz. that to which the Barometers are now brought; find the Expanfion of Air correfponding to fuch *Excefs* of Temperature by the fourth Table, which Height by Expanfion, being added to the Height already found in the 2d Table, fhews the true Height, viz. of the upper Barometer.

N. B. The 3d and laft Stage includes two Steps only, viz. 11th and 12th.

376. 11th Step. The detached Air-Thermometer *above* was — — 39½ Degrees.

The detached Air-Thermometer *below* was — — — 45

1ft. Add

1st. Add them, for the whole Heat. — — — 2)84$\frac{1}{2}$ Degrees.

2d. For *mean Temperature* of the Air-Thermometers, or a *Moiety* of the Heat, divide by 2. — 42$\frac{1}{4}$

3d. Deduct the Standard-Temperature of — — — 31$\frac{1}{4}$ from either Moiety, and the Remainder — — — 11

is the 11 Degrees of Heat, more than the Standard (*a*) for each Barometer.

For 42°$\frac{1}{4}$, and 42°$\frac{1}{4}$, equal to 84°$\frac{1}{2}$, was the whole Height of the Air at both Places of Observation in the upper and lower Stations; of which whole Height the detached or Air-Thermometer *above* received 39°$\frac{1}{2}$, and the detached or Air-Thermometer *below*, received 45°.

377. 12th Step. Find the Height corresponding to the Expansion of Air, with Excess of Heat or Temperature above the Standard-Temperature of the Barometers: and add it (as in the first Example) to the Height of the upper Barometer, corresponding to the Standard-Temperature already found in the *second* Table, and the Sum is the *true* Height of the upper Barometer.

This is to be done by referring to the 4th Table, shewing Expansion of Air with Heat; for the Application of which there are separate Instructions: see the Explanation of the 4th Table. (*b*)

378. The

(*a*) The Standard Temperature was 31°.24, which not being exactly 1 Quarter, another Decimal is added, (for Ease in Computation,) by which 31.24 becomes 31.25, i. e. by dividing one Degree of Heat into 100 Parts, and taking 25 of those Parts, or dividing the 100 by 25, the Answer is 4, i.e. $\frac{1}{4}$ of the whole 100: or (31)$\frac{1}{4}$.

(*b*) *The Foundation of the fourth Table.*
(Ph. Tr. for 1777, Part 2d, Pages 564, and 566.)—From the

378. The Expanſion of Air, in the firſt Example, is found by the 4th Table to be Feet 107.3 the *Mean* of a Series of Experiments with a Manòmeter, or Inſtrument to meaſure the *Rarity* and Denſity of the Atmoſphere, depending on the Action of *Heat* and Cold, it was found, that when the *Portion of a Tube* containing Air (at the Temperature of freezing by Farenheit, and Preſſure of $30\frac{1}{2}$ Inches (*a*) by a common Barometer) was divided into 1000 Parts; the Volume of *Air* within it, encreaſed *nearly* in a certain Proportion, as each Degree of Temperature encreaſed; viz. at a Mean, 2.43, or ſimply (by rejecting the 2d Decimal as too minute) 2.4: that is, a 1000 Parts of Air became by Expanſion with one Degree of the Thermometer, equal to 1002.43: i. e. the Portion of Air occupying 1000 Parts, did, with the Addition of one Degree of Heat, occupy 1002.43 Parts: that is (by rejecting the 2d Decimal 3 as too minute) occupied two Parts and 4 Tenths more than the thouſand.

Conſtruction of the fourth Table.

Suppoſing therefore that the Portion of the Tube containing Air, was one Foot in Length or Height, divided alſo into a thouſand Parts; one Degree of Heat woud encreaſe or expand it two Parts and four Tenths more than the thouſand Parts into which the Foot was divided.

CAUTION.

The fourth Table properly conſiſts of only nine horizontal Columns of thouſands, in Breadth: which Columns are extended in Length to one hundred Lines, correſponding to 100 Degrees of Heat.

The Table is here divided, in order that it may conform to the Size of the Pages: by which Means the Formation of each vertical Number by the following Rule, (which renders the Table ſelf-evident) might without this Caution, have been attended with ſome Difficulty.

The vertical Columns *below* the Figures expreſſing each thouſand, ſhew the Expanſion of Air *on* each reſpective thouſand, *with* the correſponding Degrees of Temperature indicated by the Thermometer in the vertical Column to the left Hand.

Example the firſt: to find the Expanſion of Air *on* one thouſand Feet, *with* one Degree of Temperature; the Anſwer in the Table is 2.4, or 2.43: i. e. 2 Feet and 4 Tenths of a Foot, rejecting the 2d Decimal as too minute.

Example the ſecond: to find the Expanſion *on* 8 thouſand Feet, *with* 99 Degrees of Heat: the Anſwer is 1924.56: and ſo of the Reſt.

Thus any of the *vertical Numbers* ſhewing the Expanſion, may

(*a*) *Theſe Experiments were made with the Manòmeter when the Atmoſphere was half an Inch heavier than in the Experiments to prove the Expanſion of Quickſilver, the Barometer then ſtanding at 30 Inches only.*

BY THE PRACTICE OF THE FIRST EXAMPLE. 301

107.3 Tenths *higher* than the 4016.8, viz. the Remainder from the 2d Table (Section 371); which Numbers added give 4124.1 Feet: viz. the true Height of the upper Station required.

CHAPTER

may be readily *formed*, by *doubling, first*, the Number immediately under each thousand in the horizontal Line, for the nine first thousands, (of which the Breadth of the Table properly consists, exclusive of the thermometric Column) for the Expansion below it; and, *afterwards*, for each Expansion immediately below the former, by adding, to the Expansion *last* found, the Number immediately under its respective thousand.

First Example: to find the vertical Number for the Expansion under the first thousand, viz. 1000, *with* 2 Degrees of Heat: the Number under 1000 is 2.43: double this: and the Answer is 4.86.

Second Example: suppose the Expansion *last* found be that *on* one thousand Feet *with* 24 Degrees of Heat; viz. 58.32: and the Expansion *on* the same thousand, *with* one Degree of Heat more, viz. on 25 Degrees, be required; add the Expansion *on* one thousand Feet, *with* 24 Degrees, viz. 58.32 to the Expansion *on* the same 1000, *with* 1 Degree, viz. 2.43

and the Answer is, by Addition, - - - - - - 60.75

Third Example: supposing the Expansion *last* found to be the Expansion *on* 9000 Feet *with* 99 Degrees of Heat, which in the Table is 2165.1.

It is required to find the Expansion *on* the same 9000 Feet, with 100 Degrees of Heat; add to the Expansion last found, viz. 2165.13, the Expansion on the same 9000 Feet, viz. 21.87 with one Degree of Heat, and

2187.00 is the Answer by Addition.

Any vertical Number shewing the Expansion may likewise *be found, first, by multiplying the first Figure, or Number, of the given thousand Feet (in the horizontal Line,) into the Answer or Expansion on the* first *thousand Feet, with one Degree of Heat: for Example;*

To find the Expansion on 9000 Feet with one Degree of Heat.

The Expansion on 1000 *Feet, with* 1 *Degree of Heat (from whence, all the other Expansions are derived) being* 2.43; *multiply that Number by* 9, *the first Figure of the given thousand Feet, and the Answer or Expansion with* 1 *Degree of Heat, is* 21.87: *hence all the Answers or Expansions,* immediately *under the horizontal Line of thousands, are* formed.

Then 2dly, *any other vertical Number or Expansion may be*
formed

CHAPTER LXXIIII.

USE AND PRACTICE OF THE FOURTH TABLE, IN THE FIRST EXAMPLE.

The USE.

Section 379. To shew in Feet, and Tenths, what is the Expansion of Air on each thousand Feet, from 1000 to 9000 Feet, *with* each Degree of Temperature from 1 to 100 Degrees, on Farenheit's Scale.

The PRACTICE.

The 12th Step applied in the first Example.

380. For the Expansion of Air with 11 Degrees of Heat on 4016.8 Feet, look in the fourth Table, *with* 11 in the left Hand vertical Column of Temperature, and (first) *on* 4000 Feet, along the upper Line: the Place of Meeting gives the Expansion of the Air, *with* 11 Degrees *on* 4000 Feet: viz. 106.92. *(a)*

Next; look *with* 11 Degrees, and (as there is a Cypher only in the Place of Hundreds) *on* 10, (viz.

formed *by multiplying the Expansion* immediately *under the* given *thousand Feet in the horizontal Line, into the* given *Number of Degrees: for Example*;

To find the Expansion on 9000 Feet, with 50 Degrees. *The Expansion with one Degree on* 9000, *is* 21.87: *therefore the Expansion with* 50°, *is* 50 *Times more, viz.* 1093.50, *and so of the Rest.*

These different Methods serve to prove the Answers, and to elucidate the Table.

(a) There is *seldom* Occasion to take more than the first Decimal out of the Table.

(viz. of the 16 Feet) call the 10, a 1000; the Place of Meeting, or Answer is 26.73:

Thirdly; *with* 11, *on* 6, (viz. of the 16,) calling it 6000; the Answer is 160.38:

Fourthly; *with* 11, *on* 8, (viz. the 8,) and the Answer is 213.84.

381. Having added the respective Expansions together, thus;

with 11°, *on* 4016.8   Feet.   Tenths.

$$\left.\begin{array}{r} 4000 = 106.92 \\ 10 = 26.73 \\ \textit{with } 11°\ 6 = 160.38 \\ \textit{on}\quad .8 = 213.84 \\ \hline \text{Expansion} \end{array}\right\} \begin{array}{l} 106.92 \\ .2673 \\ .16038 \\ .021384 \\ \hline 107.369064; \end{array}$$

(See Page 306.)

THE FOURTH TABLE,

SHEWING THE EXPANSION WITH HEAT, FROM 1 TO 100 DEGREES, ON EACH THOUSAND FEET IN THE ATMOSPHERE, FROM 1000 TO 9000 FEET.

	1000	2000	3000	4000	5000	6000	7000	8000	9000
1	2.43	4.86	7.29	9.72	12.15	14.58	17.01	19.44	21.87
2	4.86	9.72	14.58	19.44	24.30	29.16	34.02	38.88	43.74
3	7.29	14.58	21.87	29.16	36.45	43.74	51.03	58.32	65.61
4	9.72	19.44	29.16	38.88	48.60	58.32	68.04	77.76	87.48
5	12.15	24.30	36.45	48.60	60.75	72.90	85.05	97.20	109.35
6	14.58	29.16	43.74	58.32	72.90	87.48	102.06	116.64	131.22
7	17.01	34.02	51.03	68.04	85.05	102.06	119.07	136.08	153.09
8	19.44	38.88	58.32	77.76	97.20	116.64	136.08	155.52	174.96
9	21.87	43.74	65.61	87.48	109.35	131.22	153.09	174.96	196.83
10	24.30	48.60	72.90	97.20	121.50	145.80	170.10	194.40	218.70
11	26.73	53.46	80.19	106.92	133.65	160.38	187.11	213.84	240.57
12	29.16	58.32	87.48	116.64	145.80	174.96	204.12	233.28	262.44
13	31.59	63.18	94.77	126.36	157.95	189.54	221.13	252.72	284.31
14	34.02	68.04	102.06	136.08	170.10	204.12	238.14	272.16	306.18
15	36.45	72.90	109.35	145.80	182.25	218.70	255.15	291.60	328.05
16	38.88	77.76	116.64	155.52	194.40	233.28	272.16	311.04	349.92
17	41.31	82.62	123.93	165.24	206.55	247.86	289.17	330.48	371.79
18	43.74	87.48	131.22	174.96	218.70	262.44	306.18	349.92	393.66
19	46.17	92.34	138.51	184.68	230.85	277.02	323.19	369.36	415.53
20	48.60	97.20	145.80	194.40	243.00	291.60	340.20	388.80	437.40
21	51.03	102.06	153.09	204.12	255.15	306.18	357.21	408.24	459.27
22	53.46	106.92	160.38	213.84	267.30	320.76	374.22	427.68	481.14
23	55.89	111.78	167.67	223.56	279.45	335.34	391.23	447.12	503.01
24	58.32	116.64	174.96	233.28	291.60	349.92	408.24	466.56	524.88
25	60.75	121.50	182.25	243.00	303.75	364.50	425.25	486.00	546.75
26	63.18	126.36	189.54	252.72	315.90	379.08	442.26	505.44	568.62
27	65.61	131.22	196.83	262.44	328.05	393.66	459.27	524.88	590.49
28	68.04	136.08	204.12	272.16	340.20	408.24	476.28	544.32	612.36
29	70.47	140.94	211.41	281.88	352.35	422.82	493.29	563.76	634.23
30	72.90	145.80	218.70	291.60	364.50	437.40	510.30	583.20	656.10
31	75.33	150.66	225.99	301.32	376.65	451.98	527.31	602.64	677.97
32	77.76	155.52	233.28	311.04	388.80	466.56	544.32	622.08	699.84
33	80.19	160.38	240.57	320.76	400.95	481.14	561.33	641.52	721.71
34	82.62	165.24	247.86	330.48	413.10	495.72	578.34	660.96	743.58
35	85.05	170.10	255.15	340.20	425.25	510.30	595.35	680.40	765.45
36	87.48	174.96	262.44	349.92	437.40	524.88	612.36	699.84	787.32
37	89.91	179.82	269.73	359.64	449.55	539.46	629.37	719.28	809.19
38	92.34	184.68	277.02	369.36	461.70	554.04	646.38	738.72	831.06
39	94.77	189.54	284.31	379.08	473.85	568.62	663.39	758.16	852.93
40	97.20	194.40	291.60	388.80	486.00	583.20	680.40	777.60	874.80
41	99.63	199.26	298.89	398.52	498.15	597.78	697.41	797.04	896.67
42	102.06	204.12	306.18	408.24	510.30	612.36	714.42	816.48	918.54
43	104.49	208.98	313.47	417.96	522.45	626.94	731.43	835.92	940.41
44	106.92	213.84	320.76	427.68	534.60	641.52	748.44	855.36	962.28
45	109.35	218.70	328.05	437.40	546.75	656.10	765.45	874.80	984.15
46	111.78	223.56	335.34	447.12	558.90	670.68	782.46	894.24	1006.02
47	114.21	228.42	342.63	456.84	571.05	685.26	799.47	913.68	1027.89
48	116.64	233.28	349.92	466.56	583.20	699.84	816.48	933.12	1049.76
49	119.07	238.14	357.21	476.28	595.35	714.42	833.49	952.56	1071.63
50	121.50	243.00	364.50	486.00	607.50	729.00	850.50	972.00	1093.50

THE FOURTH TABLE CONCLUDED. 305

SHEWING THE EXPANSION WITH HEAT, FROM 1 TO 100 DEGREES, ON EACH THOUSAND FEET IN THE ATMOSPHERE, FROM 1000 TO 9000 FEET.

	1000	2000	3000	4000	5000	6000	7000	8000	9000
51	123.93	247.86	371.79	495.72	619.65	743.58	867.51	991.44	1115.37
52	126.36	252.72	379.08	505.44	631.80	758.16	884.52	1010.88	1137.24
53	128.79	257.58	386.37	515.16	643.95	772.74	901.53	1030.32	1159.11
54	131.22	262.44	393.66	524.88	656.10	787.32	918.54	1049.76	1180.98
55	133.65	267.30	400.95	534.60	668.25	801.90	935.55	1069.20	1202.85
56	136.08	272.16	408.24	544.32	680.40	816.48	952.56	1088.64	1224.72
57	138.51	277.02	415.53	554.04	692.55	831.06	969.57	1108.08	1246.59
58	140.94	281.88	422.82	563.76	704.70	845.64	986.58	1127.52	1268.46
59	143.37	286.74	430.11	573.48	716.85	860.22	1003.59	1146.96	1290.33
60	145.80	291.60	437.40	583.20	729.00	874.80	1020.60	1166.40	1312.20
61	148.23	296.46	444.69	592.92	741.15	889.38	1037.61	1185.84	1334.07
62	150.66	301.32	451.98	602.64	753.30	903.96	1054.62	1205.28	1355.94
63	153.09	306.18	459.27	612.36	755.45	918.54	1071.63	1224.72	1377.81
64	155.52	311.04	466.56	622.08	767.60	933.12	1088.64	1244.16	1399.68
65	157.95	315.90	473.85	631.80	779.75	947.70	1105.65	1263.60	1421.55
66	160.38	320.76	481.14	641.52	791.90	962.28	1122.66	1283.04	1443.42
67	162.81	325.62	488.43	651.24	814.05	976.86	1139.67	1302.48	1465.29
68	165.24	330.48	495.72	660.96	826.20	991.44	1156.68	1321.92	1487.16
69	167.67	335.34	503.01	670.68	838.35	1006.02	1173.69	1341.36	1509.03
70	170.10	340.20	510.30	680.40	850.50	1020.60	1190.70	1360.80	1530.90
71	172.53	345.06	517.59	690.12	862.65	1035.18	1207.71	1380.24	1552.77
72	174.96	349.92	524.88	699.84	874.80	1049.76	1224.72	1399.68	1574.64
73	177.39	354.78	532.17	709.56	886.95	1064.34	1241.73	1419.12	1596.51
74	179.82	359.64	539.46	719.28	899.10	1078.92	1258.74	1438.56	1618.38
75	182.25	364.50	546.75	729.00	911.25	1093.50	1275.75	1458.00	1640.25
76	184.68	369.36	554.04	738.72	923.40	1108.08	1292.76	1477.44	1662.12
77	187.11	374.22	561.33	748.44	935.55	1122.66	1309.77	1496.88	1683.99
78	189.54	379.08	568.62	758.16	947.70	1137.24	1326.78	1516.32	1705.86
79	191.97	383.94	575.91	767.88	959.85	1151.82	1343.79	1535.76	1727.73
80	194.40	388.80	583.20	777.60	972.00	1166.40	1360.80	1555.20	1749.60
81	196.83	393.66	590.49	787.32	984.15	1180.98	1377.81	1574.64	1771.47
82	199.26	398.52	597.78	797.04	996.30	1195.56	1394.82	1594.08	1793.34
83	201.69	403.38	605.07	806.76	1008.45	1210.14	1411.83	1613.52	1815.21
84	204.12	408.24	612.36	816.48	1020.60	1224.72	1428.84	1632.96	1837.08
85	206.55	413.10	619.65	826.20	1032.75	1239.30	1445.85	1652.40	1858.95
86	208.98	417.96	626.94	835.92	1044.90	1253.88	1462.86	1671.84	1880.82
87	211.41	422.82	634.23	845.64	1057.05	1268.46	1479.87	1691.28	1902.69
88	213.84	427.68	641.52	855.36	1069.20	1283.04	1496.88	1710.72	1924.56
89	216.27	432.54	648.81	865.08	1081.35	1297.62	1513.89	1730.16	1946.43
90	218.70	437.40	656.10	874.80	1093.50	1312.20	1530.90	1749.60	1968.30
91	221.13	442.26	663.39	884.52	1105.65	1326.78	1547.91	1769.04	1990.17
92	223.56	447.12	670.68	894.24	1117.80	1341.36	1564.92	1788.48	2012.04
93	225.99	451.98	677.97	903.96	1129.95	1355.94	1581.93	1807.92	2033.91
94	228.42	456.84	685.26	913.68	1142.10	1370.52	1598.94	1827.36	2055.78
95	230.85	461.70	692.55	923.40	1154.25	1385.10	1615.95	1846.80	2077.65
96	233.28	466.56	699.84	933.12	1166.40	1399.68	1632.96	1866.24	2099.52
97	235.71	471.42	707.13	942.84	1178.55	1414.26	1649.97	1885.68	2121.39
98	238.14	476.28	714.42	952.56	1190.70	1428.84	1666.98	1905.12	2143.26
99	240.57	481.14	721.71	962.28	1212.85	1443.42	1683.99	1924.56	2165.13
100	243.00	486.00	729.00	972.00	1215.00	1458.00	1701.00	1944.00	2187.00

Degrees of the Thermometer, from 51 to 100, on Fahrenheit's scale.

382. The decimal Points in the Anſwer muſt be changed, thus:

1. For the Place of *Thouſands* in the Queſtion, (viz. 4000,) the Anſwer muſt remain, viz. 106.92, as in the Table, which is calculated for the Place of *Thouſands*.

2. For the Place of *Hundreds*, in the Queſtion, (viz. which in the preſent Caſe was a Cypher;) if there had been a Figure or Figures in the Place of hundreds; then the decimal Point in the Anſwer muſt have been removed over *one* Figure or Place to the left.

3. For the Place of *Tens*, in the Queſtion, (viz. 10 Feet,) the decimal Point in the Anſwer, muſt be removed over *two* Figures, or Places, to the left.

4. For the Place of *Units*, in the Queſtion, (viz. 6) the decimal Point in the Anſwer, muſt be removed over *three* Figures, or Places, to the left.

5. For the Place of a *Decimal*, in the Queſtion, (viz. .8) the decimal Point, in the Anſwer, muſt be removed over *four* Figures, or Places to the left, by adding a Cypher: and for the Place of each further Decimal in the Queſtion;—*one* Place more in the Anſwer, by the further occaſional Addition of a Cypher, thus: on

Feet 4000, the Anſ. 106.92 is ſtill 106.92
   10   26.73 becomes .2673
    6   160.38   .16038
    .8   213.84   .021384
                 107.369064

383. Which Sum, by rejecting all but the firſt Decimal,

BY THE PRACTICE OF THE FIRST EXAMPLE.

Decimal, in the Answer, is Feet 107.3 Tenths equal to the Expansion of Air, *with* 11° of Heat, *on* 4016.8 Feet, the Height of the upper Barometer, with the Temperature of 31°.24, according to the 2d Table.

END OF THE LAST STAGE.

---

384. The RULE underneath, consisting of 3 Precepts *only*, is laid down by Sir George Shuckburgh, in the Transactions for 1777, Page 574, in order to ascertain the Height of Mountains, &c. (See Section 349). (*a*)

Rule copied.

385. Re-

(*a*) "R U L E.

"*Precept the* 1*st. With the Difference of the two Thermometers that give the Heat of the Barometer (and which for Distinction sake, are called the attached Thermometers) enter Table I, with the Degrees of Heat in the Column on the left Hand, and with the Height of the Barometer in Inches, in the horizontal Line at the Top; in the common Point of Meeting of the two Lines will be found the Correction for the Expansion of the Quicksilver by Heat, expressed in decimal Parts of an English Inch; which added to the coldest Barometer, or subtracted from the hottest, will give the Height of the two Barometers, such as would have obtained, had both Instruments been exposed to the same Temperature.*

"*Precept the* 2*d. With these corrected Heights of the Barometers enter Table II, and take out respectively the Numbers corresponding to the nearest Tenth of an Inch; and if the Barometers, corrected as in the first Precept, are found to stand at an even Tenth, without any further Fraction, the Difference of these two tabular Numbers (found by subtracting the less from the greater) will give the approximate Height in English Feet. But if, as will commonly happen, the correct Height of the Barometers should not be at an even Tenth, write out the Difference for one entire Tenth, found in the Column adjoining, intitled* Differences*; and with this Number enter Table* III, *of proportional Parts in the first vertical Column to the left Hand, or in the* 11*th Column; and, with the next Decimal, following the Tenths of an Inch in the Height of the Barometer (viz. the hundredths) enter the horizontal Line at the Top, the Point of meeting will give a certain Number of Feet, which write down by itself; do the same by the next decimal Figure in the Height of the Barometer*

385. Recapitulation for each Step of the Work, in the first Example; referring to the Sections.

1st. Step, in Section 353.

2d. Step, in Section 354.
Below. Barometer, Inches 29, .4 Tenths.
Attached Thermometer, 50 Degrees, Air-Thermometer 45°.

3d. Step, in Section 355.
Above. Barometer, Inches 25, .19 Tenths.
Attached Thermometer 46°, Air Thermometer, $29°\frac{1}{4}$.

From 50° subtract
46

and there remains 4 Degrees of Temperature to be added to the colder Barometer.

4th Step, in Section 356.
By Means of the first Table, find the Expansion of the *colder* Barometer, with Degrees of Heat, viz. 4° on Inches 25, .19, *gradually*, thus:
with

Barometer (viz. the thousandths of an Inch,) with this Difference, striking off the last Cypher to the right Hand for a Fraction; add together the two Numbers thus found in the Table of proportional Parts, and their Sum subduct from the tabular Numbers, just found in Table II; the Differences of the tabular Numbers, so diminished, will give the approximate Height in English Feet.

" *Precept the 3d. Add together the Degrees of the two detached or Air Thermometers, and divide their Sum by 2, the Quotient will be an intermediate Heat, and must be taken for the mean Temperature of the vertical Column of Air intercepted between the two Places of Observation: if this Temperature should be $31°\frac{1}{4}$ on the Thermometer, then will the approximate Height before found be the true Height; but if not, take its Difference from $31°\frac{1}{4}$, and with this Difference seek the Correction in Table IV, for the Expansion of Air, with the Number of Degrees in the vertical Column on the left Hand, and the approximate Height to the nearest thousand Feet in the horizontal Line at the Top; for the hundred Feet strike off one Cypher to the right Hand; for the Tens strike off two; for the Units three: the Sum of these several Numbers added to the approximate Height, if the Temperature be greater than $31°\frac{1}{4}$, subtracted if less, will give the correct Height in English Feet. An Example or two will make this quite plain.*"

IN THE FIRST EXAMPLE.   309

with 4° on 25.   = .0101   5th Step, in
with 4° on   .19 = .0000076   Section 364.
            ─────────
              25.2|
Upper Barometer, Inches 25, .2 Tenths.   6th Step, in
Lower Barometer,   -   - 29, .4   Section 366.
      End of the first Stage.
By Means of the 2d Table, find the cor-   7th Step, in
responding Heights in the Air, at 31°. 24. Section 366.
   25, .2 Answer 6225.0
   29, .4   -   -   2208.0   8th Step, in
            ─────────   Section 371.
The Remainder is   4016.8 Height in Feet, &c.
   The 3d Table, or Table for *Heights* in the At-   9th and 10th
mosphere corresponding to the *Tenth* of an Inch *on*   Steps, in Section
the Barometer, including the 9th and 10th Steps,   373.
is useless in this first Example.
      End of the Second Stage.
Detached Air-Thermometer, *above*, $29\frac{1}{2}$
Ditto -   -   -   -   -   *below*, 45°   11th Step, in
                        ─────   Section 376.
Whole Heat -   -   -   -   - 2)$84\frac{1}{2}$
Half Heat or mean Temperature $43\frac{1}{4}$
Deduct Standard -   -   -   - $31\frac{1}{4}$
                             ─────
      Moiety above Standard   11°
By Means of the 4th Table, find the Expan-   12th Step, in
sion of Air, with 11° on - - 4106.8 Feet   Section 377.
         viz.   107.3
which added to the same Height
   gives   -   -   -   -   -   4124.1 for the
true Height, in English Feet, of the *Mountain,*
or *upper Station,* sought.
         End of the last Stage.
                        CHAPTER

(310)

CHAPTER LXXV.

PRACTICE OF THE SECOND EXAMPLE:

With a diſtinct View of the Work. (Ph. Tr. for 1777, Page 579.)

Section 386. THE Point at which the Quick-silver ſtood in the Tube of the Barometer on the Mountain, or in the Car of the Balloon, being Inches 24.178 Tenths; its *attached* Thermometer, Degrees 57.2 Tenths, and its Air-Thermometer 56°; while the Barometer on the Ground ſtood at Inches 28, .1318 Tenths; its *attached* Thermometer, Degrees 61, .8 Tenths, and its Air-Thermometer 63°, .9; what is the Height of the *upper* Station?

1ſt. Step.   387. 1ſt. Step. Set down the Obſervation on the Ground, thus:

BELOW, Barometer, Inches 28, .1318 Tenths, *Attached* Thermometer, Degrees 61, .8 Tenths. *Air*-Thermometer, 63°, .9.

2d. Step.   388. 2d. Step. Set down the Obſervation, on the Mountain, or *in the Car*, thus:

ABOVE, Barometer, Inches 24, .178 Tenths. *Attached* Thermometer, Degrees 57, .2 Tenths.

3d. Step.   389. 3d. Step. From the *warmer attached* Thermometer, ſubtract the colder, thus:

$$61°, .8$$
$$57, .2$$
$$\overline{4, .6}$$

390. 4th. Step. Give the *colder* Barometer the ſame

BY THE PRACTICE OF THE FIRST EXAMPLE. 311.

same Expansion, viz. 4°, .6 with the warmer, by the *first* Table.

CHAPTER LXXVI.

PRACTICE OF THE FIRST TABLE IN THE SECOND EXAMPLE.

4th Step applied in the 2d Example.

Section 391. THE *Order* to be observed in finding the Expansion *with* 4°.6, i. e. with 4 Degrees, .6 Tenths of Heat, on 24.178, i. e. 24 Inches, .178 Tenths of the coldest Barometer. *4th Step applied.*

Find the Expansion required, thus:

Case the 1st.

1st. Part. *With* 4° *on* 24 Inches.

2d. Part. *With* 4° *on* .178 Tenths of an Inch above 24 Inches.

Case the 2d.

1st. Part. *With* .6 Tenths of a Degree, *on* 24 Inches.

2d. Part. *With* .6 Tenths of a Degree, *on* .178 Tenths above 24 Inches.

SPECIFICALLY, *thus:*

1st. Part of *Case the* 1st. To find the Expansion,

With 4° *on* 24 Inches.

2d. Part of *Case the* 1st.

With 4°, *on* .178 Tenths of an Inch above 24 Inches; begin thus:

With

With 4°, *on* 24 Inches: then,
With 4°, *on* 25: then,
With 4°, *on* 1 Inch above 24, i. e. *on* the 25th Inch: then,
With 4°, *on* .1 Tenth above 24: then,
With 4°, *on* .178 Tenths above 24.

1st Part of *Case the* 2*d.* To find the Expansion,
With .6 above 4° *on* 24; begin thus:
With 4° *on* 24 Inches: then,
With 5°, *on* 24: then,
With 1° above 4°, *on* 24, i. e. the 5th°: then,
With .1 Tenth above 4°, *on* 24: then
With .6 Tenths above 4°, *on* 24.

2d Part of *Case the* 2*d.* To find the Expansion,
With .6 Tenths above 4° of Heat *on* .178 Tenths above 24 Inches: to be done thus:

The EXPANSION *with* 4°, *on* .178 *Tenths above* 24 *Inches, being once found; divide* IT *by* 4: *and the Quotient is the Expansion with* 1° *above* 4°, *on* .178 *Tenths of an Inch above* 24 *Inches.*

Then for the Expansion with .1 *Tenth above* 4°, *on* .178 *Tenths above* 24 *Inches; add a Cypher and decimal Point to the left of the same Quotient.*

Then for the Expansion with .6; *multiply that Sum into* .6, *and add a Cypher and decimal Point.*

The Answer is the PART *of an Inch, to which* .6 *Tenths of a Degree above* 4° *of Heat, on* .178 *Tenths of an Inch above* 24 *Inches, raises the Barometer.*

It is true, the PART *is so minute as to be rejected: yet the Mode of Proceeding, in order to investigate the Expansion with Precision, is proper to be retained.*

392. PRACTICE of the first Part of *Case the* 1*st.*
For the Expansion *with* 4°, on 24 Inches;
look

look, in the firſt Table, (Sect. 363) and in the left vertical Column, *with* 4 Degrees of the Thermometer; and along the upper horizontal Line, *on* 24 Inches of Quickſilver in the Tube of the Barometer: the Point of Meeting gives the Expanſion .0097 *(a)*; which, preparatory to Addition, is to be placed under the 24, .178 thus,

.0097

PRACTICE of the 2d Part of *Caſe the firſt.*

393. In order to obtain the Expanſion, *with* 4°, of Heat *on* .178 Tenths of an Inch above 24 Inches of the Barometer; let it be conſidered where it ought to be found in the Table: for, Tenths of 1 Inch above 24 Inches, are at ſome intermediate Point between 24 and 25; that is, above 24, yet not ſo high as 25: or more than 24, yet leſs than 25.

Look therefore in the Table, *with* 4 Degrees of Heat, *on* 24 Inches; then *with* 4° *on* 25 Inches: and the reſpective Numbers are .0097 and .0101.

And by taking the Expanſion *with* 4° *on* 24 Inches, from 4° on 25; the Remainder will be the Expanſion with 4° on 1 Inch above 24 Inches, viz. on the 25th Inch, thus:

With 4° *on* { 25 = .0101 from; 24 = .0097 ſubtract:

.0004: This therefore is the Expanſion *with* 4°, *on* 1 Inch above 24 Inches.

Then *with* 4°, on .1 Tenth of an Inch above 24 Inches.

S s The

(a) There is no Occaſion to take more than four Decimals out of the Table.

PRACTICE OF THE SECOND EXAMPLE.

The Answer is the same as the former, viz. .0004, with the Addition of a Cypher and decimal Point to the left, thus; .0004 becomes .00004, viz. the Expansion *with* 4°, *on* .1 Tenth of an Inch above 24 Inches.

Then for the Expansion *with* 4°, *on* .178 Tenths, say,

If the Expansion *with* 4°, *on* .1 Tenth above 24 Inches gives .00004 Part of an Inch, what will the Expansion *with* 4°, *on* .178 give?

Thus; .1 : .00004 : : .178 ?
Multiply the two last Terms, thus:

```
        .00004
         .178
        ──────
        00032
        00028
        00004
        ──────
       0000712
```

: and, as in Multiplication of Decimals, the Product must have as many decimal Places, as are in the Factors; a Cypher must be added to the left Hand, thus: .00000712: but having divided that Product by the first Term .1, viz. a Decimal, the Answer is a Cypher less; viz. .0000712.

This Answer is the Expansion *with* 4°, *on* .178 Tenths of an Inch above 24 Inches: prepare it for *Addition*, as the former, 24.178
       .0097
       .0000712

PRACTICE of the first Part of *Case the 2d.*

394. For the Expansion of .6 Tenths of of a Degree of Heat, (more than the 4 Degrees) on 24 Inches of the *coldest* Barometer; it should
           be

PRACTICE OF THE SECOND EXAMPLE. 315

be confidered where fuch Tenths can lie in the Table.

Now .6 Tenths of 1 Degree, (more than the 4°) are at fome intermediate Point of the Thermometer between 1 and 2 Degrees: above 1; yet not fo high as 2: or more than 1; yet lefs than 2.

Therefore .6 Tenths of 1 Degree above 4 Degrees, are fomewhere between the 4th and 5th Degree: above 4; yet not fo high as 5: or more than 4; yet lefs than 5.

Look in the Table (Section 363); firft *with* 4 Degrees of Heat, *on* 24 Inches, and then *with* 5 Degrees of Heat *on* 24 Inches; and the refpective Numbers are .0097 and .0121: and by taking the Expanfion *with* 4 Degrees *on* 24 Inches, from the Expanfion *with* 5 Degrees *on* the fame 24 Inches; the Remainder will be the Expanfion *with* 1 Degree above 4° *on* 24 Inches: viz.

$$\text{with } \begin{cases} 5° = .0121 \\ 4° = .0097 \end{cases} \text{ on 24 Inches, as in whole Numbers.}$$

Remainder, .0024

This therefore is the Expanfion *with* 1 Degree of Heat, above 4, viz. *with* the 5th Degree, *on* 24 Inches of the Barometer.

Then fay, if 1 Degree of the Thermometer (above 4, viz. the 5th Degree) gives by Expanfion, a certain additional Height, or Part of an Inch, viz. .0024, *on* 24 Inches of the Barometer; what Height will 6 Degrees give? Anfwer 6 Times *more*.

Multiply the 2d and 3d Terms, and divide by the firſt, thus;

$$1 : .0024 :: 6?$$
$$6$$
$$\overline{.0144}$$

is the Expanſion, or Height, in Parts of an Inch, for 6 Degrees.

And farther, to proportion for the Decimal; ſay as .1 Tenth of a Degree gives a certain Tenth of the former .0024, in additional Height, viz. .00024; what Height will .6 Tenths give? Anſwer, .00144.

Prepare this *Height* for Addition to the Numbers already found.

PRACTICE of the 2d Part of *Caſe the* 2d.

395. To find the Expanſion of .6 above 4° on .178 above 24 Inches.

The Expanſion *with* 4° *on* .178 is already found to be .0000712: divide it by 4, and the Anſwer is .0000178, viz. the Expanſion *with* 1° *on* .178 above 24 Inches:

And, for the Expanſion with .1 Tenth; the Anſwer, with the Addition of a Cypher and decimal Point to the left, becomes .00000178.

Laſtly, for the Expanſion with .6, ſay,

$$\text{If } .1 : .00000178 :: .6?$$

Multiply the 2d and 3d Terms, and divide by firſt:
$$.00000178$$
$$.6$$
$$\overline{.000001068.}$$

The Anſwer is a Decimal leſs, viz. .00001068; i. e. the Decimal of an Inch, to which .6 Tenths of a Degree above 4 Degrees of Heat, on .178

Tenths

PRACTICE OF THE SECOND EXAMPLE. 317

Tenths of an Inch above 24 Inches, raises the Barometer: which, after all, is so inconsiderable, that it may be fairly rejected.

Yet the Rules by which these Deductions are made, may be useful in other Cases.

Prepare for Addition, as before.

The Decimals, in the Answers, may be omitted, when they exceed four Places.

396. 5th Step. To proceed with the second Example. *5th Step.*

Place the different Expansions now found, above each other, Units, Tens, &c. under Units, Tens, &c. preparatory to Addition, thus:

For the Expansion *with* 4°, .6 *on* 24, .178:

1st. *with* 4°,	*on* 24,		.0097
2d. *with* .6	*on* 24,		.00144
3d. *with* 4°,	*on*	.178	.0000712
4th. *with* .6	*on*	.178	.00001068

The Expansions with 4°, .6 added = .01122188
To the Sum add the Height of
   the *colder* Barometer - - 24.178

                                24.1892|

The Answer is Height of the *colder* Barometer, now equal in Temperature to the *warmer:* (rejecting all but the four first Decimals.)

397. 6th Step. Place the Barometers *now* of the same Temperature, i. e. *equal* to the warmer, in one View, thus: *6th Step.*

    1st. the *upper* Barometer,   24.1892
    2d. the *lower* Barometer,   28.1328

The 7th Step applied in the second Example.
398. Find the Height, in Feet, in the 2d Column *7th Step.*

lumn of the 2d Table, corresponding to Inches and Tenths of the *upper* barometric Tube, in the 1st. Column of the same Table, thus: (Sect. 371.)

The Barometer standing at 24.1892; it must be considered where, in the 2d Column of the 2d Table, a Height corresponding to *such* Inches and Tenths can lie: and the Answer is, somewhere *above* 24 Inches .1 Tenth, but not so high as 24 Inches .2 Tenths: 24 Inches .1892 Tenths, being *more* than 24 Inches .1 Tenth, but *less* than 24 Inches .2 Tenths.

First then, look in the 1st Column for Inches 24, .1 Tenth; and the corresponding Height in Feet is 7388.0: but the Height for 24, .2, in the 2d Column, beneath the former Number, is *only* 7280.1.

8th Step. 399. 8th Step. Subtract the latter from the former and the Remainder is 107.9, the same as in the 3d Column: viz. the Height, in Feet and Tenths, corresponding to one Tenth only, namely, the 2d Tenth above Inches 24, .1 Tenth: with the Temperature of 31.24 of Farenheit, for which sole Purpose the 2d Table is calculated.

A new Question *then* arises, viz. what are the Heights in Feet and Tenths, corresponding to the remaining Tenths or Decimals of an Inch above Inches 24, .1 Tenth,

viz.   .08
                  .009
                        .0002 ? which is to be resolved, by Application of the 3d Table, or Table for *Tenths*, which see, (Section 373.)

APPLICA-

APPLICATION OF THE TABLE FOR TENTHS. 319

400. *9th Step applied in the 2d. Example.* 9th Step.
First for the *upper* Barometer.

Look in the Table for Tenths, in the left vertical Column with 107, (rejecting the .9, as too minute;) and along the horizontal Line at the top, with 8: and find the Answer *gradually*, thus:

1st. With 107, and 8, (as a whole Number,) answering to .08: which, in the Place of Meeting, gives 86 Feet.

2d. With 107, and 9, (as a whole Number,) answering to .009: which, in the Place of Meeting, gives 7.

3d. With 107, and 2, (as a whole Number,) answering to 0002: which, in the Place of Meeting, gives 21.

Place them in View, and add, and bring them back again into Decimals, thus:

With 107 and 8, answering to .08 giving 86. Feet
- - and 9, - - to .009 - - 9.7
- - and 2, - - to .0002 - .21
                                    ─────
                                    95.9|1

(Next: with the 9, *if required*; which was before rejected:) but there being no .9 Tenths in the left Vertical, call it 90, and allow for it in each Answer by moving the decimal Point two Places to the left, thus: with

90, and 8, answering to .08 giving 72 = .72
and 9, - - - to .009 - 81 = .081
and 2, - - - to .0002 - 18 = .0018
                                    ─────
                        To .8|00|28
Add the former Sum 95.9|
                                    ─────
              Total = 96.7)
                                Which

Which 95.9 is the *Height* in Feet and Tenths corresponding to .0892 Decimals of an Inch above Inches 24 .1 Tenth: and 24 .1 gave Feet 7388.0 in *Height*; therefore an additional *Height*, of so many Tenths of an Inch of Quicksilver in the Tube of the Barometer, must give in Feet, a *less* Height of the Barometer elevated above the *imaginary* Level indicated at 32 Inches.

10*th. Step*. 401. 10th. Step. Subtract the *Height* in Feet, corresponding to the *Expansion* on .0892 Tenths of an Inch, *(less* than Inches 24.2 Tenths, of the *upper* barometric Tube,) from the *Height*, in Feet, corresponding to *the Expansion on* Inches 24.1 Tenth of the same barometric Tube, continuing at the Standard Heat, *(a)* viz. 7388.0

95.9
———

The Remainder 7292.1 gives the real, viz. the *less* Height of the *upper* Barometer, at 24.1892 with the Standard Temperature.

Repeat the same Process, viz. the 9th. and 10th. Steps, for the *lower* Barometer, thus:

For the lower Barometer in the 2d. Example.

First, Find the Height, in *Feet*, of the lower Barometer, standing at Inches 28.1318 Tenths, in the 2d. Column of the 2d. Table, corresponding to Inches and Tenths of the Quicksilver in the barometric Tube, in the first Column of the same Table, thus:

The lower Barometer standing at 28.1318; it must be considered, where in the 2d. Column of the 2d. Table, a Height corresponding to such Inches and Tenths can lye: and the Answer is, somewhere above 28 Inches, .1 Tenth, but not so

---

(a) See Section 368, Note *(a)*.

PRACTICE OF THE SECOND EXAMPLE. 321

fo high as 28 Inches .2 Tenths : 28.1318 Tenths being more than 28 Inches .1 Tenth, yet lefs than 28 Inches .2 Tenths.

First, then, look, in the firft Column for 28.1, and the correfponding Height, in Feet, is 3386.6: but the Height for 28.2, is only - - 3294.0: fubtracting the lefs from the greater; the Remainder is - - - - - - 92.6, the fame as in the 3d. Column, viz. the Height, in Feet and Tenths, correfponding to *one Tenth only* above 28.1.

Having therefore found that Feet 92.6 Tenths, are the Height, correfponding to one Tenth only above Inches 28.1 Tenth, of the lower Barometer, with the Temperature of freezing; for which *fole* Purpofe, the 2d Table is calculated;— a new Queftion arifes, viz. what are the Heights, in Feet and Tenths, correfponding to the remaining Decimals above 28.1, viz.

.03
.001
.0008; to be refolved by Application of the third Table, or Table for Tenths, which fee, (in Section 373.)

Look in the 3d. Table, with 92, (omitting the .6 as too minute) and with

3 anfwering to .03, which gives 28 =Feet 28.
1 - - - to .001, - - - 9 = - - .9
8 - - - to .0008, - - - 74 = - - .74
—————
29.6|4

Which 29.6 is the *Height* in Feet and Tenths correfponding to .0318 Tenths above Inches 28.1 Tenth : and Inches 28.1 Tenth gave Feet 3386.6
T t   Tenths

Tenths in Height: therefore an additional Height of so many Tenths or Decimals of an Inch of Quickfilver in the Tube of the Barometer, muſt give in Feet, a *leſs* Height of the *lower* Barometer, elevated above the *imaginary* Level indicated by the Quickſilver reſting in the Tube at 32 Inches.*(a)*

402. Therefore ſubtract the *Height*, in Feet, correſponding to the *Expanſion on* .0318 Tenths of an Inch *(leſs* than Inches 28.2 Tenths of the *lower* barometric Tube,) from the Height, in Feet, correſponding to the *Expanſion on* 28.1 Tenth of the ſame Barometer, viz.

$$3386.6$$
$$29.6$$
———

and the Remainder - 3357.0, gives the *real* Height in Feet of the lower Barometer, at 28.1318 when above the *imaginary* Level, and with the Temperature of *freezing* by the ſecond Table.

403. Then, by taking the Number of Feet and Tenths *above* the imaginary Level, (indicated by the Quickſilver, in both Tubes, reſting at 32 Inches) anſwering to the *Expanſion on* Inches and Tenths of the *lower* Tube, from the Number of Feet, &c. by the former Proceſs, anſwering to that of the *upper* Tube; viz.

upper 7292.1
lower 3357.0
———

and the remaining Feet 3935.1 Tenth is the *Height*, by which the *Station* of the *upper* Barometer exceeds the *Station* of the *lower*; both be‐
ing

(a) Section 368, Note *(a)* on Note *(a)*.

PRACTICE OF THE SECOND EXAMPLE. 323

ing at the Temperature of 31°.24 on Farenheit's Scale. See Section 371.

END OF THE SECOND STAGE.

Section 404. 11th Step.   *11th Step.*
(See the Practice in the 1st Example, Sect. 376.)
*Air-*Thermom. ABOVE was 56°.
*Air-*Thermom. BELOW was 63. 9

Whole Heat	119. 9 (0 adding a Cy-
Half Heat	59. 95 [pher)
Standard-Heat	31. 24
which deduct; and there	
remains each Moiety,	28. 71
above the Standard-Heat.	

405. 12th Step. (See the Practice in the first *12th. Step.* Example, Section 377.)

By the fourth Table, find the Expansion of Air, *with* 28.71, (more than the Standard-Temperature) *on* Feet 3935, .1 Tenth, gradually, thus:

406. *First, with* 28° *on* Feet 3000 = 204.1 *(a)*
        900 as 9000 = 612.3
         30   3000 = 204.1
          5   5000 = 340.1
         .1   1000 = 68.0

Note: 1st. The decimal Point in the Answer corresponding to the Place of *Thousands*, in the Question, is to remain, as taken from the Table calculated for thousand Feet, thus: 204.1.

T t 2   2d. For

2d. For *Hundreds* in the Queſtion, remove the decimal Point *one Place* in the Anſwer, thus: 612.3 becomes 61.23:

3d. For *Tens*, *two* Places, thus: 204.1 becomes 2.041:

4th. For *Units*, *three* Places, thus: 340.1 becomes .3401:

5th. And for each *Decimal*, a Place more, by adding Cyphers to the left, if wanted, thus: 68.0 becomes .00680.

407. Place the plain and decimated Anſwers, in one View, and add the latter together, thus:

$$204.1 = \text{the ſame } 204.1$$
$$612.3 = \text{becomes } 61.23$$
$$204.1 = - - - 2.041$$
$$340.1 = - - - .3401$$
$$68.0 = - - - .00680$$

viz. Expanſion of Air with
28° on 3935.1 - - $\Big\}$ 267.7|179

408. *Second*, with .71° on Feet 3000 = 517.5
$$900 \text{ as } 9000 = 1552.7$$
$$30 \quad 3000 = 517.5$$
$$5 \quad 5000 = 862.6$$
$$.1 \quad 1000 = 172.5$$

In order to decimate theſe Anſwers, it muſt be obſerved that the Expanſion was not *with* 71 Degrees, but with .71 *Tenths* of a Degree of Heat; therefore the decimal Point correſponding to 3000 Feet in the Queſtion, muſt in the Anſwer be removed *two* Places to the left, thus: 517.5

becomes

(a) Taking one Decimal *only* out of the Table.

PRACTICE OF THE SECOND EXAMPLE.

becomes 5.175 : for the 100, three Places : for
1.5527   the 10, *four* Places : and so
.05175   on.
.008626
.0001725
―――――――
6.7|882485

The Expansion with .71 being found, viz.
Feet 6.7 Tenths; add it to the Expansion on
28 Feet already found, viz.
267.7
―――――
274.4 Answer.

Which *Height* in Feet and Tenths, corresponding to the *Expansion* of Air with 28°.71 Tenths of a Degree of Heat more than the Standard 31°.24, being added to the *Height* in Feet and Tenths, corresponding to the *Expansion on Inches* of the Quicksilver in the *upper* Barometer, with the Standard-Heat, already found, viz.   3935.1
gives the *real Height* of the *Moun-*   274.4
tain, or *upper Station*, sought.   ―――――
                                          4209.5

END OF THE THIRD STAGE.

―――――――――

The second Example briefly *stated: referring to the Sections.*

409. Below: Barometer 28.1318.
Attached Thermometer 61°.8; Air ditto 62°.9.
Above: Barom. 24.178.
Attached Thermometer 57°.2; Air ditto 56°.
Degrees of Heat, viz. 4 .6 to be added to

the

RECAPITULATION OF THE SECOND EXAMPLE.

Section, 391. the *colder* Barometer at Inches 24.178 Tenths, by the firſt Table, viz.   .0112
Parts of an Inch of the Quickſilver in the Barometer, raiſed by $4°.6$ of Heat. ———
    The Sum   24.1892
is the POINT, in Inches and Tenths of an Inch, at which the upper Barometer *now* reſts, being of *equal* Heat with the lower.

End of the firſt Stage.

Section, 399. By the 2d. Table, find the *Height*, in Feet and Tenths, correſponding to the *ſaid* POINT when at the Standard - Heat; gradually, thus: the *Height* correſponding to Feet 24.1 is 7388.0: then with the Difference 107.9, (rejecting the .9)

Section, 400. Find the Height by the 3d. Table correſponding to   .08   86.0 ⎫
          .009   9.7 ⎬ = Feet 95.9 Tenths.
          .0002   .2 ⎭

Which Height ſubtract from 7388.0
                           95.9

And there remains, in Feet,   7292.1

The Height correſponding to Inches 24.1892 Tenths of the *upper* Barometer, with the Standard Temperature of 31.24; for which ſole Purpoſe the 2d. Table is calculated.

Repeat the laſt Proceſs with the *lower* Barometer, reſting at 28.1318, gradually, thus:

Section 401. By the 2d. Table, find the *Height* correſponding to 28.1, which is 3386.61; then with the Difference 92.6 (rejecting the .6) find the correſponding *Height*, by the 3d. Table for the remaining Tenths or Decimals of an Inch, above 28.1, viz.
                                            .03

RECAPITULATION OF THE SECOND EXAMPLE.

$$\left.\begin{array}{ll}.03 & 28.0 \\ .001 & .9 \\ .0008 & .7\end{array}\right\} = \text{Feet } 29.6 \text{ Tenths.}$$

Which *Height* subtract from 3386.6   Section 402.
                               29.6

And there remains, 3357.0 viz. the *Height* in Feet corresponding to Inches 28 .1318 Tenths of the lower Barometer, with the Standard Temperature of 31.24, for which sole Purpose the 2d. Table is calculated.

Subtract the *Height* in Feet, corresponding to   Section 403. Inches of Quicksilver in the upper Barometer, viz. 7292.1 from ditto in *lower* Barometer, viz. 3357.0 and there remains the *Height* in Feet
——— of the upper Barometer at the Stan‑
viz. 3935.1 dard‑Temperature of 31.24.

End of the second Stage.

On which Number of Feet, viz. 3935.1, by the   Section, 404. 4th Table, find the *Height*, with 28°.71 of Heat:

With 28°.   *on* Feet 3935.1 = 267.7 and
With   .71 *on* the same   = 6.7

                  Sum   274.4 : which Height, more than the Standard‑
Heat, being *added* to   -   -   3935.1
the Height, with the Standard, ———
gives the true Height, viz.   4209.5.

End of the third Stage.

CHAPTER

(328)

CHAPTER LXXVII.

PRACTICE OF THE THIRD EXAMPLE,

REFERRING TO THE SECTIONS. (a)

Section 410. *BELOW*: Barom. Inches 30, .0168 :

Attached Therm. 60°.6 ; Air-ditto, 60°.2 :

Above: Barom. - - Inches 29, .5218 :

Attached Therm. 56°.6 ; Air-ditto, 57°.

Subtract the *colder* ——— from the *warmer*, and there remains 4° of Heat to be added to the *colder* Barometer ; to give it an *equal* Temperature : which is to be done by *the 1st Table*, thus :

Section 356. To find the Expansion *with* 4° of Heat, *on* the *colder* Barometer ; (which, as before, is the *upper* Barometer) standing at Inches 29, .5218 Tenths.

First, *with* 4° on 29 Inches=.0117 :

2d, *with* 4° on .5218 Tenths *above* 29 Inches :

In order to obtain which, begin

          with 4° *on* 29 = .0117

    then *with* 4° *on* 30 = .0121

Subtract for the Expansion *with* ———

4° *on* 1 Inch above 29, and there

remains - - - - - - .0004.

Then

(a) THE QUESTION : In the upper Gallery of the Dome of St. Peter's Church at Rome, and 50 Feet below the Top of the Cross, the Barometer, from a Mean of several Observations, stood at Inches 29.5218 Tenths : the attached Thermometer being at Degrees 56.6 Tenths ; and the Air-Thermometer at 57 Degrees : at the same Time that another, placed on the Banks of the River Tyber, one Foot above the Surface of the Water, stood at 30.0168, the attached Thermometer at 60°.6, and the Air-Thermometer at 60°.2 : what was the Height of the Building above the Level of the River ?

PRACTICE OF THE THIRD EXAMPLE.   329

Then for the Expansion *with* 4° *on* .1 Tenth Section 362.
of an Inch above 29 Inches ; add a Cypher and
decimal Point, viz.   .00004 :

Then for the Expansion on .5128, multiply Section 363.
the two laſt Terms, and divide ─────
the Product by the firſt Term
.1 : the Anſwer is ‑ ‑ ‑ .0002|0872
Add the Expanſion *with* 4° *on*
  29 Inches, juſt found, ‑ .0117
to the Inches of the *colder*
  Barometer, ‑ ‑ viz. 29.5218
                          ─────────
          Anſwer ; Inches 29.5337 Tenths of
the *colder* Barometer, are *now* expanded equally
with the *warmer* : (rejecting the Decimals as in
Section 395.)

Place the Barometers, thus :
  Upper Barometer,   29.5337
  Lower Barometer,   30.0168
    End of the firſt Stage.

411. *By the* 2d *Table*, and in the 2d Column, Section 371.
find the *Height* of each Barometer, *with* the
Standard-Heat, in Feet and Tenths, correſpond‑
ing to the Inches and NEAREST Tenth *above*
and *below* the Point required : and
  Firſt of the *upper*, at 29.5337 :
  The Inches and *neareſt Tenth* is above
              Feet.
  29.5, correſp. to 2119.7⎫ Difference
and below 29.6, cor. to 2031.5⎬ between .5 and .6
              ──────   ⎭ above 29 Inches.
                88|.2

412. *By the* 3d *Table*, *with* the *Difference* 88 Section 373.
            U u   Feet,

Feet, find the *Expansion* on the remaining Decimals, above 29.5, viz. on .0337, thus:

on 03 = 26 decimated 26.
003 = 26 - - - 2.6
0007 = 62 - - - .62
                                      —————
                                Feet 29.22

From the *Height* corresponding to   29.5
viz. Feet 2119.7 Tenths,
subtract the   29.22, i. e. Height cor. to   .0338
and there ————   ————
remains   2090.4|8, the *Height* cor. to 29.5338
with Expansion of the Standard-Heat.

413. Repeat the 4 last Steps for the *lower* Barometer, at 30.0168.

1st. The Inches and *nearest* Tenth is *above*
     30. corresp. to Feet 1681.7 ⎫ Difference of
and *below* 30.1 cor.   -   1595.0 ⎬ .1 above 30
                               ——— ⎭ Inches.
                               86|.7

2d. Then with 86 Feet, find the *Expansion* on the remaining Decimals, above 30,
viz. .0168, thus: on 01 = 9 - 9.
006 = 52 - 5.2
0008 = 69 - .69
                                      —————
                                Feet 14.89

414. (3d.) From the *Height* corresponding to 30 Inches, viz. Feet 1681.7 Tenths,
subtract the Height   14.89 corresp. to .0168,
                         ————————
and there remains 1666.8|1, the Height corresp. to 30.0168, with *Expansion* of the Standard-Heat.

                                          4. From

PRACTICE OF THE THIRD EXAMPLE. 331

4th. From the *upper* Height, at 2090.48
Subtract the *lower* Height, at   1666.81

And there remains the Height 423.67 in Feet and Tenths of the upper Barometer, with the Standard Temperature.
      End of the second Stage.

415. Detached Therm. *above* 57°   Section 374.
     Detached ditto, *below* 60.2
        Whole Heat - - 117.2
        Half Heat - - 58.6 (0 adding a
        Standard Heat - - 31.24 [Cypher)

which being deducted, leaves 27°.36, viz. Degrees of Heat more than the *Standard*, for each Barometer.

416. By the 4th Table, find the Expansion of Section 380.
Air, with 27°.36, on Feet 423.67 Tenths.

First, with 27°, *on* 423.67, thus :   Section 406.
viz. *on* 400 as 4000 = 262.4 decimated 26.24
      20 as 2000 = 131.2 - - - 1.312
       3 as 3000 = 196.8 - - - .1968
      .6 as 6000 = 393.6 - - - .03936
     .07 as 7000 = 459.2 - - - .004592
            Expansion = 27.692752

Second, with .36 *on the same*, thus :   Section 407.
on 400 as 4000 = 349.9 decimated .3499
      20 as 2000 = 174.9 - - - .01749
       3 as 3000 = 262.4 - - - .002624
      .6 as 6000 = 524.8 - - - .0005248
     .07 as 7000 = 612.3 - - - .00006123
          Expansion = .37050003
      Add the former 27.692752
      Height in Feet 28.06325203

    U u 2   418. Which

417. Which Height for Expanfion of Air, *with more than* the Standard Heat, being ADDED *(a)* to the Height, for Expanfion of the Barometer, *with* the Standard-Heat, gives the true Height of the upper Barometer, at the given Heat.

For *Expanfion* of *Air* above Standard Heat,
      Height in Feet 28.0
For *Expanfion* of *Barometer*,
 with Standard : Height in Feet 423.6

418. True Height of the *upper* Barometer 451.6
Lower Barometer 1 Foot above the Water 1.0
Height of the Top of the Crofs above the
 Gallery - - - - - - - - 50.0

Height of the Top of the Crofs above the
 Tyber - - - - - - - - 502.6
Height of the fame, meafured the fame
 Day geometrically, was - - Feet 502.9

    End of the laft Stage.

         CHAPTER

(a) See Section 375. 2dly. If the Moiety, *Half-Heat*, or mean Temperature of the Air, *is equal* to the Standard-Temperature, to which the two Barometers are brought, by the 2d Table; the fourth Table, for *Expanfion of Air*, is needlefs : the Height already found, in the 2d Table, being the *true* Height of the *upper Station*.

3dly. If the Moiety, *Half-Heat*, or mean Temperature of the Air, is *lefs than* the Standard-Temperature of 31°.24; fubtract the mean Temperature from 31.24; and with the Remainder find the Expanfion, as ufual, by the 4th Table : fubtract the Sum, (which is a correfponding Height in Feet and Tenths) from the Height in Feet and Tenths of the *upper* Barometer, at the *Standard-Temperature*, in the 2d Table : and the Remainder will be the *true* Height of the *Mountain* or *upper Station*. Section 384, Note *a*.

CHAPTER LXXVIII.

**PRACTICE OF THE FOURTH EXAMPLE, *(a)*
FOR MEASURING SMALL HEIGHTS.**

Section 419. Attached Therm. *below*, 71°.0
Attached Therm. *above*, 70 .5

Subtract, and there remains - - .5

Tenths of a Degree of Heat to be added to the *colder* Barometer (which in the present Case is the *upper*, but might possibly have been otherwise) by the 1st Table.

By this Example, *small* Heights are easily measured.

First, with 0°.5 *on* 29 Inches. To obtain which, begin
    with 1°.0 *on* 29 Inches = .002 :
    with 0°.1 above 1°, *on* 29 = .0002 : then
    with 0°.5 above 1°, *on* 29 = .001.

Prepare it for Addition to the *colder* Barometer.
colder Barometer - - - - 29.985
Expansion *with* .5 above 1°, *on* 29   .001
                                            29.986

Secondly, with .5 Tenths above 1°, *on* .985 Tenths above 29 Inches. To obtain which, (having already found the Height from Expansion *with* .5 above 1°, *on* 29 Inches, to be .001;) since the Expansion on .985 Tenths above 29 Inches, is somewhere above 29, yet below 30 Inches;

(a) THE QUESTION: Near the Convent of St. Clare, in a Street called *La Strada dei Specchi*, at Rome, the *lower* Barometer stood at 30.082, its attached Thermometer 71 Degrees, and detached ditto at 68 Degrees: on the Tarpeian Rock, or West-End of the famous Hill called The Capitol, the *upper* Barometer was at 29.985, its attached Thermometer 70°.5, and detached ditto 76°: what was the Height of the Eminence?

Inches; find the Expansion *with* .5 above 1°, *on* 30 Inches, thus:

 firſt, *with* 1°, - - - *on* 30 = .003
 2d. *with* 0°.1 above 1°, *on* 30 = .0003
 3d. *with* 0°.5 above 1°, *on* 30 = .0015

Subtract the Expansion *with* .5 Tenths above 1°, *on* 29 Inches, from the Expansion *with* .5 Tenths above 1°, *on* 30 Inches:

  viz. on 30 = .0015
    on 29 = .001

The Anſwer is - - .0005, the Height from Expansion, *with* .5 Tenths above 1°, *on* 1 Inch above 29, i. e. on the 30th Inch: Then, if 1 Inch above 29 gives .0005; .1 gives .00005:

      and   985

multiplied	00025
as whole	00040
Numbers,	00045

    give - .0004|925
 add the former Number 29.986
and, for the three remaining Decimals, *may* be ſubſtituted 1 Decimal in the fourth Place -   1

colder Barometer of equal Heat ⎱ 29.9865
with the *warmer* - - - ⎰

420. *When the Quickſilver in each Barometer indicates the ſame Number of Inches*, differing *but one or two Tenths at the moſt*; (*which will frequently be the Caſe, in levelling flat Countries, or meaſuring ſmall Heights*;—*inſtead of the uſual Method, (to find the Height of each Barometer* ſeparately, *with the Standard-*

FOR MEASURING SMALL HEIGHTS.   335

Standard-Heat, by the 2d Column *of the* 2d *Table, as in Section* 411;)—*it will be more convenient,*

1st. *To subtract the lower Barometer from the upper. Then,*

2dly. *By the* 3d Column *of the same Table, find the* DIFFERENCE, *(viz.* of one *or* two Tenths *at the most)* below *the Inches and* nearest Tenth *of the lower Barometer.*

And lastly, *with that* DIFFERENCE, *find by the* 3d Table, *the Height at the Standard-Heat, corresponding to the remaining Decimals above the upper Barometer.*

421. (1*st.*) From the lower Barom. viz. 30.082
    Subtract the upper - 29.9865
Remaining Decimals *above* the upper .0955

2*d.* Find, by the 2d Table, the Height corresponding to the Inches, and *nearest* Tenth *above* and *below* the Point at which the Quicksilver rests in the lower Barometer.

The Inches and *nearest* Tenth is
 above 30 Inches, correspond. to Feet 1681.7
and *below* 30.1, coresponding to - - 1595.0
             86.7

which is the DIFFERENCE of .1 *below* 30.1.

Lastly. Find, by the 3d Table, *with* the DIFFERENCE, viz. 86 Feet, *on* the remaining Decimals, for the Height, in Feet, corresponding to the Standard-Heat.

  viz. .09 - - 77 - = 77. Feet.
    .005 - 43 - = 4.3
    .0005 - 43 - = .43

  Answer, Height in Feet 81.73
corresponding to .0955 above Inches 29.9865
              Tenths

Tenths of an Inch, of Quicksilver in the upper Barometer thus brought to the Standard-Heat.

422. Prepare for Expansion of Air from Excess above Standard-Heat, on the same Number of Feet:

Detached Thermom. *above* 76°.
Detached Thermom. *below* 68.0

	Whole Heat	- -	144.0
	Half Heat	- - -	72.0 (0 adding a
	Standard-Heat	-	31.24 [Cypher]

which deduct, and there remains - - - - - - 40.76: with which, by the 4th Table, find the Expansion of Air on Feet 81.73:

First, with 40°, *on* 81.73, thus:

on 80.	as 8000	-	777.6	=	7.776
1.	as 1000	-	97.2	=	.0972
.7	as 7000	-	680.4	=	.06804
.03	as 3000	-	291.6	=	.002916
					7.944156

Second, with .76 *on* 81.73, thus:

on 80.	as 8000	-	1477.4	=	.14774
1.	as 1000	-	184.6	=	.001846
.7	as 7000	-	1292.7	=	.0012927
.03	as 3000	-	554.0	=	.0000554

Expansion .1509341
add the former Expansion - - 7.944156

Sum of the Expansions, viz. Height in Feet - - - - - - } 8.0950901

from Excess of Heat above Standard, *with* 40.76 *on* 81.73,

ADDED

PRACTICE OF THE FOURTH EXAMPLE. 337

Added to the Height at the Standard-Heat, in Feet ⎬ 81.73
gives, in Feet and Tenths, the true ―――
Height of the Tarpeian Rock   89.8|2.

CHAPTER LXXVIII.

A CALCULATION TO ASCERTAIN THE HEIGHT OF THE BALLOON ON THE DAY OF ASCENT: ONE BAROMETER AND ONE THERMOMETER ONLY, BEING TAKEN UP INTO THE CAR.

Section 423. THE Question is stated from Section 36: and the Mode of Operation taken from the *Recapitulation* of the second Example, Section 409.

Observation before the Ascent:

Below: Barometer 29.8; attached Thermometer 0; detached Thermometer 65°.

Above: Barometer $23\frac{1}{4} = 23\frac{25}{100}$ or 23.25 (*a*); attached Thermom. 0; detached Thermom. 65°.

There being no attached Thermometers; the *first* Table is useless: the Barometer below is therefore supposed to be of the same Temperature as when above; the detached Thermometer remaining at the same Degree, viz. 65°.

State the Barometer, thus: when *below*, at 29.8
when *above*, at 23.25.
End of the first Stage.

424. Find the Height (at the Standard-Heat) corresponding to the Inches and *nearest* Tenth above and below 23.25: i. e. above 23.2, and below 23.3: by the 2d Table.

X x   Now

(*a*) Sadler's *Practical Arithmetic*, Page 293.

Now 23.2 corresponds to 8379.7: and the Difference of .1 above, i. e. to 23.3, is in Feet =112|.1: by the 3d Column of the same Table.

With this Difference, consult the 3d Table: i. e. with 112, (omitting the .1 as too minute) on the remaining Decimals above 23.2, viz. on 05, as on 5, or $\frac{5}{10}$; and the Answer is 56 Feet: which Number being subtracted from 8379.7, the Remainder 8323.7, is the Height in Feet of the Barometer in the Car, at the Standard-Heat.

Repeat the last Process for the Barometer on the Ground.

Now 29.8, by the 2d Table, corresponds to 1856.0; and there being no Parts or Decimals more minute than a Tenth, viz. .8, there is no Occasion for the 3d Table.

Subtract the Barometer in the Car, from the same when on the Ground; and, by the 2d Table, upper Barom. 23.25, corresp. to 8323.7, and the lower Barom. 29.8, - - - - to 1856.0: the Remainder is the Height in Feet ——— of the Barometer in the Car - viz. 6467.7, with the Standard-Heat.

End of the second Stage.

425. Detached Therm. above, at 65°
Detached Therm. when below, at 65

    Whole Heat   -   -   -   130
    Half Heat   -   -   -   65.(00 adding
    Standard-Heat   -   -   31.24 [Cy-
    ——— [phers)

which deduct, and there remains 33.76 Degrees more than the Standard-Heat, for each Barometer.

Then for the Expansion of Air, with such Heat more than the Standard, consult the 4th Table,

HEIGHT OF THE BALLOON MEASURED.

Table: viz. *with* 33°.76 *on* Inches 6467.7, the Height of the Barometer in the Car with the Standard-Heat, thus:

426. *First, with* 33°, *on* 6467.7

on 6000 as 6000=481.1, decimated 481.1
    400 as 4000=320.7 - - -   32.07
     60 as 6000=481.1 - - -   4.811
      7 as 7000=561.3 - - - - .5613
    .07 as 7000=561.3 - - - - .05613
                Expansion=518.59843

427. *Second, with* .76 *on* 6467.7:

on, as before, 6000=1108. decim. 11.08
          4000= 738.7 - - .7387
          6000=1108. - - .1108
          7000=1292.7 - - .012927
          7000=1292.7 - - .0012927
              Expansion=11.9437197
       Add the former 518.59843
      Total Expansion=530.5|542197

viz. Height *by Expansion* in Feet, with more than the Standard-Heat, add to Height in Feet at the Standard-Heat - - - - 6467.7

428. The true Height, in Feet and Tenths, of the Barometer in the Car - - - - - - - - 6998.2

       Feet in a Yard 3)
    Yards in a Mile 1760)2332.2 Feet.
                   1760 (1 Mile.

Yards in a Quarter of a Mile 440) 572(1 Qr.
                    440
                    32 Yards.

The Height of the Balloon 1 Mile, 1 Quarter, 32 Yards, and 2 Feet.

*End of the laſt Stage,
and of the Menſuration of Heights.*

N. B. A *thermometric* ſliding Rule, for the Expanſion of Quickſilver, and of Air, may poſſibly, from the foregoing Tables, be ſo contrived and adapted to the Barometer, as to tell the Height by Inſpection, while in the Car of the Balloon.

CHAPTER LXXX.

HINTS, ON THE CHEAPEST METHOD OF INFLATING BALLOONS, WITH DESCRIPTIONS OF DIFFERENT MODELS FOR A GASS-STEAM-ENGINE.

Section 429. THE *Expence* attending the Inflation of Balloons is a ſolid Objection to their frequent Uſe.

A Check is thereby given to every Improvement that might otherwiſe be expected from a Repetition of Experiments.

It is, in ſhort, the chief Difficulty under which the AIRONAUTIC ART at preſent labours.

This Difficulty, however, if once overcome, (and of which there is little Doubt) will probably bring thoſe extraordinary Machines, into general Eſtimation.

What *now* coſts fifty Pounds, may *then* be done for five: abating the Expence of the preparatory Engine.

Monſ. Lavoiſier, by the Application of Steam to Iron Filings encloſed in a Copper Retort, has generated

generated inflammable Air, or light Gafs *(a)*: and Dr. Prieftley, by converting a Gun-Barrel into a Steam-Engine, has produced a Gafs 13 Times lighter than common Air; *(b)* whereas by the prefent expenfive Method, with Metal and Acid, the Gafs for Inflation is feldom more than fix Times lighter.

What has hitherto been atchieved on a fmall Scale, is here meant to be extended.

As no Particulars are made public, or at leaft, have yet come to the Author's Knowledge, relative to the Conftruction of fuch a Gafs-Steam-Engine, as may, with Safety and Effect, be applied to the Inflation of Balloons; the following Defcriptions of different Models may deferve fome Notice :—may poffibly excite the Attention of the Ingenious ; and put them on contriving *eafier* Means to obtain the *fame* End.

I.

430. Let there be an Iron *Hot-hearth*, one Yard fquare, and two Inches thick. Let it be *fet* on a common Brick Stove, built as near the Ground as poffible, (or even below it) in the open Air. Its Chimney to confift of malleable Iron, flat at the Top, and ftrong enough to fupport a Tea-Kettle or Boiler to produce Steam : and extending at leaft one Yard from the End of the Hearth horizontally, before it turns up. It may rife three or four Yards high, flanting farther from the Hearth : the Form a hollow Cylinder : with a Turn-Cap at the Top, two Feet long,

fet

(a) The Writer has not hitherto been fo fortunate as to meet with the original Memoir, containing the Particulars of this curious Experiment by Monf. Lavoifier.

(b) Dr. Prieftley's Experiments and Obfervations relating to Air and Water. Ph. Tr. for 1785, Vol. 75, Part 1, Page 279.

set on at right Angles; for the Management of the Smoke.

Suppofing then the Fire-Place to face the Weft; the Chimney may project Eaftward. The North Side is to be appropriated to the Iron-Borings or Turnings; and on the South Side is to be depofited the Drofs or Calx.

A Muffle or Mould of malleable Iron is to be fcrewed and luted over the hot Hearth. The four Sides of the Muffle next the Hearth are to have horizontal Lips or Rims projecting half an Inch: and Screws are to be driven, throu' Holes drilled at proper Diftances, into the Hearth. The Sides are to rife upright a Couple of Inches: clofing, as they rife, in the Form of a hollow Cylinder, one Foot in Diameter, and perhaps a Yard above the Hearth: which is now converted into a *Gafs-Steam-Engine*.

It is propofed to ftrew over the *Hot-hearth* a thin Layer of Borings, one Tenth of an Inch thick; to which Layer when *red* hot, the boiling Steam is to be applied. The extricated Gafs is to be conveyed from the Top of the Cylinder, by Means of an extended Trunk of Tin, and varnifhed Linen, into a Tub of cold Water kept *continually* flowing over, into which a few Lumps of quick Lime are thrown: and from thence the Gafs is to rife into the Balloon.

431. The Iron, whether Filings or Turnings, proper for Inflation, muft be *bright*; wholly free from Chips, Bits of Wood, and all heterogeneous Particles: but particularly RUST, and GREASE: *lefs* than a cubic Inch of the latter, woud fpoil a Ton of the brighteft, and otherwife the beft prepared Materials. (Section 339.)

A

A Day or two *only*, before a Balloon is inflated; the proper Quantity of bright Iron fhoud be heated RED HOT in *Charcoal*, and fuffered to go cold.

For Want of this fimple Preparation of the Iron, the Gafs has proved defective in Point of LEVITY: altho' the Balloon appeared fully inflated.

This Misfortune happened at Birmingham, and other Places.

432. The *Defideratum* is, *quickly* to apply, and *remove* the Borings, keeping the Machine *nearly* Air-tight. For, it is *now* well known, that the Gafs will *explode*, if one-third Part of common Air be introduced: or, if lefs; it may *unite* with the *Gafs*, and detract from *its* Levity.

433. The following *Particulars* may likewife be confidered as an Improvement.

II.

1. To lay a Plate of Iron, Brafs, or Copper, over the Hearth; which, if made of *caft* Iron, will be apt to crack, in Contact with the Steam; and will alfo unite with and concrete the Iron Turnings or Gun-Borings into a folid Mafs, that woud be feparated with Difficulty.

2. To make the Drofs-Pit in the Form of a hollow Wedge, narrow at the Top: fcrewing and luting it to the South Side of the Hearth. It fhoud hold the Drofs arifing from a Ton of Borings; which will be fufficient for the Inflation of a Balloon, to carry one Perfon.

3. On the North Side is to be erected a Platform of Brick, a Yard fquare, *floored* with a Plate of Iron: the infide Surface to be even with the Bottom of the Hearth.

4. The

4. The Ton of Borings is to be placed on the *Floor*, and covered with another Muffle, fecured and luted to the Side of the Hearth: having a Communication of two Inches high, and one Yard wide, with the Bottom of the Hearth: as the Drofs-Pit has.

5. A Brafs or Copper Rake is to remain within the two Muffles: to prefs forward the Borings, fpread them over the Hearth; ftir them frequently;—by turning the Inftrument, fcrape them into the Drofs-Pit; and apply frefh from the *Depofit*.

6. To perform thefe manual Operations within the Machine kept Air-tight; it will be neceffary, at the exterior End of the Muffle, to faften a ftrong leathern Cafe, made very wide and pliant, and two Yards long: into which the End of the Rake-Handle is to be inferted.

III.
434. *The Mode of Operation.*

The Borings being fpread on the Hearth, and *red* hot; the Steam Pipe is to be opened, and *inftantly* fhut. The Gafs being *fuddenly* extricated; the Pipe is to be opened, and fhut again as before: the Borings pufhed into the Drofs-Pit, and a frefh Supply fpread. This Procefs to be renewed, till the Inflation is completed.

If it be thought neceffary to prevent the Steam from communicating with the whole Depôt of Borings, and fo evolve too much Gafs; a little Brafs Door with Hinges of the fame, might be made to hang from the Top of the Communication between the two Muffles: which Door opening inwards, and hanging vertically,

WITH GASS PROCURED BY MEANS OF STEAM. 345

tically, woud by the Preſſure of the Gaſs, ſtop up the Open: and yet, if made ſtrong, *not* prevent the Operations of the Rake, at proper Times.

IIII.

435. The Machine woud be leſs complex, with one large Muffle, ſomewhat longer North and South than the Hearth; furniſhed with leathern Caſe and Rake. Put in the Borings at one End: keep the Steam-Pipe always open; with a *Hand* at the Rake; puſhing away the Droſs, and preſſing forwards freſh Borings.

V.

436. Further: it has ſince occurred, that a Machine in the Form of a GUN-BARREL, *extended in all its Dimenſions*, will probably anſwer *every* Intention.

And of this Kind are the hollow cylindrical Tubes, of *different* Lengths, and about a Foot in Diameter, (*a*) which are *caſt*, for the Conveyance of Steam, from the Boiler of a Steam-Engine.

Such a one, (previouſly lined with a Cylinder of Copper, or malleable Iron, to prevent the Adheſion of the Borings, when reduced to a Calx by the Admiſſion of Steam;) might be placed horizontally over a Stove, (with or without a Chimney) and ſurrounded with *red* hot Coals.

The Ton of Borings might be depoſited at one End of the Tube; and, by Means of the Air-tight flexible leathern Caſe, be preſſed with a Rake, *gradually* into the Fire, and *beyond* it when calcined.

Care muſt be taken to make the *Apparatus* nearly Air-tight.

(*a*) The Diameter may be enlarged.

The Steam fhoud pafs into the Tube, from *below:* and the Gafs be conducted towards the Balloon throu' another Iron Cylinder, nearly equal in Diameter and at right Angles with the firft; lying alfo in an horizontal Direction; along the Ground.

The Tubes might be *forged* or *caft,* fo as to form but one rectangular Piece.

The further End of the fecond Tube fhoud communicate with a *third,* made of Tin, and bent downwards about a Foot; thence at right Angles, for fix Inches: then to rife up, alfo at right Angles, the Length of fix Inches more.

The Tin Tube is to defcend into a Ciftern of cold Water, made to flow over continually, by a frefh Supply; and into which, a few Lumps of Quicklime fhoud be thrown.

The Gafs, which will prefs upwards throu' the Water, is to be received into an inverted Funnel, and thence (as in Section 339, Art. 2.) conveyed to the Balloon.

VI.

437. The following Alterations woud fuperfede the Ufe of the Rake, and *leathern* Cafes: the latter of which, by any accidental Crack or Flaw in the Leather, might admit a fufficient Quantity of common Air to produce an Explofion.

The cylindric Form of the Copper, or malleable Iron (to be ufed as a Lining for the Tube) is to be changed, into that of a half Cylinder, or inverted Muffle: and to be perforated with fmall Holes.

This Muffle is to be *nearly* filled with a Ton of Iron Borings: (the Ends to be made up, to prevent the Borings from falling out into the Tube;)

Tube;) the Muffle itself is to be supported by a Cradle (*a*) of the same Form, made of STRONG Copper Wire, (*b*) like the *open Iron-Wire*-Fenders: and the whole is to be thrust into the Tube.

The Length of the Muffle depends on the Quantity of Borings that are intended to be used.

The Ends of the Tube shoud not be made so strong as the Tube itself: that, if an Explosion happens, they *may* give way first, and prevent a Rupture of the Tube: not that any Danger is to be apprehended, that such an Event will take Place, so long as the Steam-Pipe is attended to, by a proper Person: the above Caution being only given, to prevent a Possibility of Rupture.

Each End shoud be cast, or forged with a hollow Handle; and shoud screw into the Tube.

The Length of the Tube shoud be such, that the Person who attends the Steam-Pipe, shoud feel no Inconvenience from the Heat of the Fire.

Nine Feet woud therefore be a proper Length: the conducting Tube the same.

Within six Inches from each End of the Tube which holds the Borings, a Hole, half an Inch in Diameter shoud be drilled across the Middle of the Tube, in an horizontal Direction.

Into these, an Iron Axis is to be fitted, (so as to take out *occasionally*) and pass throu' the Tube: each End of the Axis is to project outwards a Couple of Inches, and to be made *square*, for the Socket of a strong Iron Winch or Handle.

Each

(*a*) By Means of the Cradle, *both* are more easily moved: the Muffle is prevented from adhering to the Tube; and Steam is admitted to the Borings.

(*b*) Copper sustaining a *red* Heat, better than Iron; the latter of which, *calcines* with Steam, or, in cooling.

Each Axis to be furnished with a strong Chain, of equal Length with the Tube; one End of which Chain is to be riveted, or otherwise fixed, to the Middle of the Axis; and the other, to be fastened *occasionally* to one Extremity of the Cradle and Muffle: the second Axis and Chain in like Manner, to the other Extremity.

The Muffle is to be placed in the Cradle: both are then to be thrust into the Tube, and fastened to the Chain at the farther Axis: in which Position the Muffle may be filled with Borings, and gradually drawn into the Tube; till the same End has reached the Center of the Fire. The nearer End is then to be hooked by the nearer Chain, already wrapped round the nearer Axis: and the light Iron Caps to be screwed on each End of the Tube.

438. The Boiler for Steam may be fixed on any Part of the Tube near the Fire, and near the opposite Axis; so that one Person may attend both the Steam-Pipe, and Axis. The Steam to be conveyed throu' a small Orifice made in the Bottom of the Tube, between the same Axis and the Fire.

439. As soon as the Materials, above the Center of the Fire, are supposed to be *red* hot, the Steam-Pipe is to be opened for a Moment and SHUT AGAIN. The extricated Gafs will be instantly HEARD, rushing throu' the Vessel of *cold* Water; and as instantly SEEN to swell the varnished Linen-Trunk as it passes into the Balloon.

The Steam-Pipe is to be regulated by these infallible Signals: and the Process continued, till that Quantity of Borings, that was in the Center

Center of the Fire, and consequently *red* hot, is supposed to be calcined.

At which Time, the Handles are to be applied to the Axis, and the Cradle and Muffle drawn 5 or 6 Inches forward into the Fire.

When drawn, too far; Recourse must be had to the second Axis.

440. If great Expedition is required, two or three Conductors from the same Tube may be used: and, at the Distance of six or seven Feet from the Fire, *Tin-Conductors* may be added; taking Care that they are *made*, *applied*, and *continued Air-tight*.

T H E E N D.

An *alphabetical* INDEX of the CONTENTS:

Referring to the SECTIONS and NOTES, but *not* to the *Pages*.

A.

	Section.
Absorption of Water by Air, *Experiment to prove* the.	247
Accumulation of Air, *mediocèanal*.	259, 260
Aërial Scenes *described*.	39, 47, 51, 56
Air gives FORM to *Things*.	53
- gentle, its Effect on the *Surface* of the Balloon.	201
- calm, its *Effect* on the *Surface* of the Balloon.	202
- pure, cool, defloguifticated, perpetually defcending.	252
- *defcending Torrents* of, on Etna and Teneriffe.	265
- *Reception* and *Difperfion of*, what.	280
Air-Bottle-Balloon, *its Ufe*.	311
- - - preferred to an *interior* Balloon.	314
Aironaut *Employments* of the, in the Balloon.	29
- - *Attitude* of the, in the Balloon.	32, 33
- - *loft over a Country* well-known when *below*.	177
- - to *try* different Heights, to find a *favourable Wind*.	309
- - to *wait*, in the *Calm above* the Clouds, for a Wind.	309
Airoftat, a fmall one *firft* liberated.	8
Altitude *apparent*, from the Balloon when *ftationary*.	49
- - barometric.	49, *b*
Anchor and Cable.	13
Apogay Winds, what.	241
Apparent Height *proportioned* to the *barometric* Height.	49
Appearance of a Plain *below*, the Size of a moderate Carpet, what.	179, 189
Appearance of a Plain *below*, the Size of a Handkerchief, what.	181, 187
Appearances at *different Altitudes, from the Balloon*.	213
Articles, *Weight* and *Number* of.	26
Afcent, to *check* and *promote*.	14
- - Preparations for.	22
- - of the Balloon at 40 Minutes paft I. o'Clock.	28
- - with *twenty Pounds* of *Levity*.	28
- - of Balloons, Caufes to *limit* the.	279
- - *proper Times* for.	285
- - *new* Mode of, to *determine* the *Height*.	299

Atmofphere

AN INDEX OF THE CONTENTS:

                                                                                          Section.

Atmosphere *gross*, when seen throu', *from below*. - 55
  - - Depression of the. - - 232
  - - State of, *favorable* to the *Direction* of Balloons. 268
  - - Conjectures concerning the *Warmth* of the *superior*. - 275
  - - probably *respirable* at great *Altitudes*. - 277
  - - Height of. - - - - 290
  - - Weight of, in *England*. - - 290
Attention to the Balloon *necessary*. - - 35
Aurora Borealis, Conjectures concerning the *Appearance* of. 274

B.

Ballast of what it consisted. - - 27
  - - when to be *first* thrown out. - - 21
  - - in Hand, ready to throw out. - - 91
  - - thrown down. - - - 67, 95
  - - thrown over *nearly* 32 Pounds. - - 103
  - - poured down at once 20 Pounds. - 183
Balloon going to Sea. - - 75, 87, 90
  - - in a quiescent Bed of Air. - - 75
  - - of rowing it to any Point, in a Calm. - 75
  - - drawn aside out of the Perpendicular. - 103
  - - shrunk to its former Shape. - 123
  - - alternately rising and falling. - 125, 138
  - - in the Air five Hours and a Quarter. - 207
  - - sustained above Water, how. - 294, 295
  - - best Form of. - - - 307
  - - Double, what. - - - 314
Balloons their Defects, and further Improvements. 303
  - - Air-tight Varnish for. - - 320, 325
Barometer, and Thermometer, when stationary. - 36
  - - Fluctuation of the Quicksilver in the. 37
  - - Mensuration of Heights by the. - 350
Beautiful preferred to the Sublime, in Prospects. - 42
  - - Appearance. - - - 43
Bladders necessary. - - - 26
  - - began to *crackle*. - - 116
Bottles of Air thrown down, Caution. - 74, 77, 84
Breath not affected, nor visible, during the Excursion. 126
Breeze Sea-. - - - 88, 92, 257

C.

Cable, and Anchor or *Grapple*. - - 13
  - - to be fastened to a *Center above* the Car. - 297
                                                                  Calculations

	Section.
Calculations of the *Distance* seen from the Balloon.	52, *a*.
- - of the Height of *Mountains*.	171, *a*.
Calm *above*, and Wind *below*, at the same Time.	168
Canal artificial, Duke of Bridgewater's, Appearance of.	166
Cannon first discharged at IX. o'Clock.	7
- - the second Time, at XII.	11
- - the third Time, at 40 Minutes and a half past I.	64
- - the last Time, at 10 Minutes and a half past II.	62
Car and Hoops, their *Dimensions*.	35
Caution to keep the Circle clear during the Inflation.	23
- - against the *Dropping* of Water *out of* the Balloon.	31
- - on Landing.	98
- - *not* to open the upper Valve.	122
Charts Balloon, first suggested.	168
Chilliness *first* perceived, 92; again.	109
- - *felt* near moist Places.	283
Circularity of Prospect.	79, 221
Circumstance, *each* to be recorded.	4
Circumstances apparently *superfluous*, mentioned and repeated, why.	5
Clouds, an upper Tier *seen* to move in a safe Direction.	7, 46
- - Perspective of the.	51
- - *appearing* in rapid Motion.	163
- - View of the, taken from above them.	130, 171
- - Colouring of the.	172
- - *highest visible*.	213
Cochuc-Varnish.	320
Cold, its Effects on the Balloon.	94
Colour of the Rivers, red.	44
- - of the City of Chester, *blue*.	45
- - of Thunder-Clouds.	54
- - of upper Clouds.	57, 172
Colours, *primary*, of Objects beneath.	129
Columns of Air, depressing, observed by the Ancients.	239
Compass, the properest Kind of.	38, *a*.
Conclusions, useful.	159
Conjunction of the Planets *preceding* a Hurricane.	211
Contemplation of the Prospect.	113
Course of the Balloon traced, to shew the Manner in which it was affected in passing over Water.	78
Curls and Streams of Air, Smoke and Vapour.	250, *b*.
Currents of Air, horizontal.	20
- - from *above*, to be guarded against.	21

Z z   Currents

AN INDEX OF THE CONTENTS:

	Section
Currents *under*, of Air.	87
— — of Air, blowing *to and from* great Towns.	250
— — of Air, *contrary*, at different Heights, at the same Time.	267
— — the Balloon rising throu' *different*.	106

D.

Defects in the Composition for Balloons, *remedied*.	320
Depressing Torrents of Air.	254
Depression of the Atmosphere.	232
— — over *moist* Places in *fair* Weather.	243
— — of the Atmosphere proved from History.	253
— — *nocturnal*, of the Atmosphere.	267
— — corroborating Proofs of a.	268
Depth below, conveys no Idea of Distance.	157
Depths, Mensuration of, with Barometers, &c.	348, 368, a, a.
Descent of the Balloon, to *retard* the.	15
— — Signs of the.	17, 159, 181
— — at *first rapid*, with a rushing Noise.	96, 97
— — Proof of *gentle*.	100
— — Change in *visible* Objects, during the.	182
— — of Balloons over Water, *enquired* into.	229, 230
— — — — — Means to prevent.	294, 295
Description of the Ascent.	47
Diameter of the Prospects *above* and *below*.	52, 79
Diminution of Objects, *excessive*, when seen from the Balloon.	223
— — — — Laws respecting the.	224
Direction of the Balloon, Hints for the.	315
Distance seen from the Balloon, Calculations of the	52, a.
— — of the Balloon from *Chester*, at the Report of the 4th Cannon.	64
— — Idea of, from *Experience*.	158
— — what is the *greatest*, to be seen from the Summits of the *highest* Mountains.	171, a.
— — at which an Object can be distinguished by a *good* Eye.	175, a.
— — of the Balloon-*Course*.	191
— — at which, the Balloon was seen.	227
— — and Height of a Balloon, found by a Quadrant.	310
Dove turned out of the Car.	61

E.

Earth removed from *Sight*.	170
Echo	

		Section.
Echo none *above*.		39
Eknêfiai Winds, what.		241
— — a dry Wind.		267
Electricity of the Air.		65
Elliptic Solid, the Form of the Balloon an.		160
Employments of the Aironaut.		32
Engines *Steam*, Models of, for Inflation, described		429
Equatorial Hoop, its Use.		161, 315
Evaporation of *Steam*.		249
Expansion of the Balloon, by what Manouvre.		132
Experiment to prove whether the *superior* Atmosphere be *hazy*, tho' the Sun continue *shining*.		47, *a*.
Experiments necessary, in order to improve the Modes of *Direction*.		296
Examples in the Mensuration of *Heights* with Barometers. See Table.		
Example 1st, Practice of the.		351
— — — Recapitulation of the.		385
— — 2d, Practice of the.		386
— — — Recapitulation of the.		409
— — 3d, Practice of the.		410
— — 4th, Practice of the, to determine *small* Heights.		419
— — 5th, Practice of the, to determine the Height of the Balloon.		423

F.

Fish *Diodon-Globe*, a *Model* for Balloons.	377
Flag *white*, hung out a Quarter of a Mile in Length.	4
— — hung out half a Mile, in all.	66
— thrown *down* at a Mile high.	59
— Descent of the.	60
— *white*, its Effect on the Balloon.	70
— — Progress of the Balloon marked by the	91
— — *impeding* the Balloon.	103
— — the remaining one unfolded.	105
— — shewed a Change in the *Direction* of the *Wind*.	105
Flights with the Balloon, for three Hours longer.	193
Flying-Coach.	149
Foot Roman, the *Measure* of a.	49. *b*.
Form of the Balloon at its *greatest* Altitude.	14
— — — the *same* at each Descent.	159

G.

Gas not offensive during the *Voyage*, why.	34
— procured by Means of *Acid*.	338

Z z 2   Gas

	Section.
Gafs procured by Means of *Steam*.	429
Geography Balloon, *firſt* ſuggeſted.	167
Globe-Fiſh, a *Model* for Balloons.	377
Grapple or Anchor.	13
Gums Copal, Sandarac, Maſtic, &c.	326

H.

Heat of the *Sun, greateſt*, while in the Car.	59
Height *apparent*, proportioned to the *barometric* Height.	49
— of the Balloon, when *ſtationary*, at the *firſt* Aſcent, viz. 2332 Yards	52, *a*.
— in the Balloon, conveys no Apprehenſion of falling.	156
— of *principal* Mountains, noted.	171
— of a Mountain, ſeen at a *Diſtance*, calculated.	171, *a, a*.
— to which Balloons will *probably* aſcend.	278
— fixed, Method of aſcending to any.	299
— of the Balloon, to aſcertain by a *Quadrant*.	310
— *preparatory* Inſtruments to obſerve the.	350
— of the Balloon meaſured.	425
Heights to meaſure, Denſities to eſtimate.	299
— of the Atmoſphere, while they encreaſe in an *arithmetical* Progreſſion, the Denſities are ſaid to encreaſe in *geometrical* Progreſſion: the Meaning of ſuch Terms.	301, *a*.
Hemiſphere *upper only*, of a Balloon to be inflated.	315
Hoop equatorial, its Uſe.	161, 315
Horizontal Motion, Signs of, *deceitful*.	18
Hours proper for the Aſcent of *Balloons over Water*.	254, 255, 261
Hygrometer *Horſe-Hair*, the *beſt* Kind.	217

I.

Illuſtration of the Scenery.	72
Improvement during the Proceſs of Inflation.	24
Improvements how to be made in the propulſive Machinery.	319, 330
— — in the Proceſs of Inflation by Acid, ſuggeſted.	339
— — ſuggeſted in the Proceſs by Steam.	429
Incorrectneſs of Maps.	81
Inflation began at X. o'Clock, with a ſmall Balloon.	8
— — Degree of, to be limited.	278, 317
— — Proceſs of.	339
— — by Means of Acid, Expence ſaved in the.	347
— — by Means of Steam, Expence ſaved in the.	429

Inflation

	Section.
Inflation by Means of Steam, Model and Mode of.	429
- - by Steam, preferred to the Process by Acid.	429
Information derived from the Shape of the Balloon,	159, 160
Inventory of the Voyage.	12
Iris 1st, round the Shadow of the Balloon.	56
- 2d.	73
- 3d.	136
Iron *bright* and *fresh*, proper for Inflation.	431

L.

Landing, Manouvres during the.	98
- - first, near *Frodsham* in *Cheshire*.	100
- - second, near *Warrington* in *Lancashire*.	188
- - Precautions to secure a safe.	297
- - in *windy* Weather, Precautions to secure a safe.	298
- - *improved* Mode of.	317
Latitudes variable, *light Airs* playing in Eddies, common in the.	241
Level of the *lowest* Stratum of Clouds in *fair* Weather.	93
- all Inequalities of Surface reduced to the *same*.	111
Light of a *red* Colour, Conjectures concerning the.	222

M.

Machinery *propulsive*, to be used in the *Calm, above Winds*.	319
Magnitude of Objects, Laws respecting the.	224
Manouvres seen at a *great* Distance.	140
Map consulted.	174
Mast, a light *hollow*.	315
Meanders of the River *encreased* to the *View*.	81
Mensuration of Heights and *Depths* by Barometers.	348
Methods to ascertain the *true* Height.	350
Method, the cheapest to inflate by Steam instead of Acid.	429
Mistakes to be noticed, to prevent Repetition.	2
Motion encreased, progressive not perceived.	165
Motion of Air, called *Reception and Dispersion of Air*, what.	280
Mountains, Names and Heights of principal.	171, a.
- - their Use.	265
Mouth of the Balloon, *closed*.	102

N.

Neck of the Balloon, how to place it.	31
- - *first* tyed.	102
- - risen near *eight* Feet upwards.	119
- - an *Attempt* to reach it.	121
- - held *Air-tight* in the *Hand*.	125

Notes

AN INDEX OF THE CONTENTS:

                                                            Section.

Notes made during the Voyage.   36

O

Objects diminishing as the Balloon arises, Description of. 109
Objects, all *terrestrial*, disappearing.   163
Order preserved during the Inflation.   23

P.

Parashute or Umbrella.   15
        the Balloon formed a vast.   184
Perspective new.   39, 229
Place where the Balloon alighted.   100, 187
Points, the plainest generally most essential, frequently overlooked.   4, 338
Preparations for Ascent.   22
Prospects *most beautiful*, at what Height.   93
      below noted.   128
Pulley or Reel.   13

R.

Rain *warm* in Winter, accounted for from the Theory of Accumulation.   270
Reception and Dispersion of Air.   280
Reel or Pulley, its Defects remedied.   41 *a*.
Respiration easy during the Excursion.   114
Resistence of the Air, as the *Square* of the Velocity of the falling Body.   15 *a*.
Rising, Signs of.   16, 30
Rivers, no *Appearance of* Water in the.   110
Rule, general for measuring Heights, copied.   384
Rusty Iron, *improper* for Inflation.   398

S.

Sail, three seen in the *Liverpool* Channel.   108
   - *triangular* Latteen, *purposely to retard* the Balloon. 315
   - Anemometer, what.   315
   - Weights to be added to the.   316
   - Vane, what   318
Scenes aërial, described. See Sublime.
Sea-Breeze discovered.   88
   - its Duration.   256
   - its Extent.   257
Sensation of *rising* described.   30
Sensations accompanying the Balloon.   141, 154
Shadow of the Balloon *traced* on the Clouds. 56, 73, 136
                                                 Shadows

REFERRING TO THE SECTIONS.

                                                          Section.

	Section
Shadows, their Length, *at Noon*, calculated.	84
— — — at half past III. calculated.	100
— — encreased, seemed to raise the Objects.	127
Shape of the Balloon *altered*.	118
Sign of Descent.	181
Signs to be observed in the Management of Balloons.	14, 15, 17, 20
Situation novel, peculiar to the Balloon.	221
Sound of the Gass throu' the upper Valve.	134
— in the Air, an *uncommon*.	162
Sounds immediately under the Balloon, their Effects.	175, a.
Spirits raised by the Purity of the Air.	155
Spunges of Air.	247
Squalls of Wind, the Day preceding the Ascent.	6
Stationary, the Balloon.	36, 122
Steam, Mode of Inflation by Means of.	429
Storms of *Collection* and *Dispersion*.	232, 263
Sublime and beautiful Scenes.	3, 39, 47, 48, 49, 51, 71, 84, 112
Sun, when hottest.	59
Sympathy of the Spectators.	46

T.

Table the 1st. See Mensuration.	
— — for Expansion with Heat, from 1 to 40 Degrees, on Inches of the Barometer, from 9 to 32 Inches.	363
— the 2d, shewing the Variations of the Barometer, at each Inch and Tenth of the Quicksilver, from 1 to 32 Inches, the Air being at the freezing Point.	371
— the 3d, for easy Calculations, from the 2d Table.	373
— the 4th, shewing the Expansion with Heat, from 1 to 100 Degrees, on any Number of Feet in the Air.	381
Tastes not altered, on Account of the Height.	65
Thermometer warmer *above* than *below*.	126
Thermometers compared.	12, c.
Thunder-Clouds described.	52
— — — under the Balloon.	172
Tide of Air in the Atmosphere.	291
Tides highest.	288, 289
Time, noted.	7, 8, 11, 22, 28, 36, 62, 63, 68, 73, 77, 85, 100, 101, 124, 162, 174, 186, 203, 206
— of Ascent.	28

Time,

AN INDEX OF THE CONTENTS:

                                        Section.

Time, in which the Excursion was performed, viz. two Hours and a Quarter. - 191
— Noon, a dangerous one, for Balloons to pass an Arm of the Sea. - - 256
— the best, pointed out. - - 256
— Noon and full Tide, improper: Midnight and low Water, proper Hours for Ascent, over Water. - - - 287
Torrents of Air medioceanal, depressing. 257, 258, 259
— — — — — accumulating. - 260
Transparency circular, of Vapour. - - 222
Twine cut, lest it should prove a Conductor of Electricity between the Balloon and Earth. 103

U.

Useful Conclusions. - - - 159
Utility of Balloons. - - 332, 333
Utility *general*, of Balloons. - - 338

V.

Valve upper, emits the *lightest* Gas. - - 124
— *first* tried. - - - 133
— -Swing, or Umbrella-Pendulum, as *propulsive* Machinery, communicates a *progressive* Motion to the Balloon. 319
Vane-Sail. - - - - 318
Vapour, Observation of the *reddish*. - - 33
— *white, beautiful* Effects of. - - 71
— — began to be accumulated at a *certain* Height. 80
Vapours, their *Transparency*. - - 222
Varnishes. - - - 320, 325
Velocity of the Balloon. - - - 192
Vessels, the *four* and the River Wever *disappeared*. 110
View *circular*, from the Balloon at its *greatest* Elevation. 55
— of the Balloon over *Helsbye-Crag*. - -. 77
— of the Clouds, *from* above *them*. - - 171
— *from* the Balloon of the Country between Chester and Rixton-Moss. - - 192
Vis Inertiæ. - - - 70, 316

W.

Warmth of the superior Atmosphere. - 275
— of the Air above Plains and cultivated Countries. 276
— of the Air over the *Sea*, at certain Times and Seasons. - - - 276
— descending from *above*. - - 284

Water

Section.

Water poured down, to observe the Effects of Air upon it.	74
— Balloon influenced on its Approach to.	76, 78
— Balloon above the Influence of.	131
— the Descent of Balloons over.	229
— the Causes of their Descent over.	230
— Absorption of, by Air.	247
— a curious Phenomenon seen on its Surface.	249, 250, b.
— Means to prevent the Descent of Balloons over, and within its Influence.	294, 295
Waves of Air.	21
— of the Sea, the Dashing of, heard; the Sea being invisible.	80
Weather, about the Time of the Excursion.	211
Weighing during the Inflation avoided, how.	24
Weight of Provisions and Articles.	24
— of the Balloon, and its Apparatus.	25
Wind heard below.	86
Winds, the Eknèfiai and Apogay, what.	241
— the Directions in which they blow.	253, a.
— the Eknèfiai productive of Cold.	253, a.
— Land- and Sea-.	253, a.
— contrary, at different Heights, their Use to waft Balloons to a given Point.	268
Wings, their Use, first to retard, second to direct.	315
Winter-Dress, preparatory.	26, 338
— -Prospect from the Balloon.	169

www.ingramcontent.com/pod-product-compliance
Lightning Source LLC
Chambersburg PA
CBHW032030220426
43664CB00006B/425